NEUTRAL OR BETTER

How to always feel content about your life no matter what disaster you are standing in

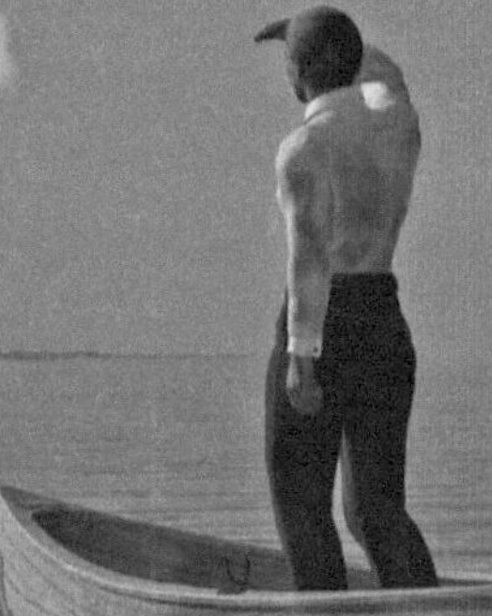

DOUGLAS MAZELL

Author of The Teenager's Crystal Ball

NEUTRAL OR BETTER

How to always feel content about life no matter
what disaster you are standing in

A guide for easy mental stability for every day of life.

Neutral or Better

How to always feel content about life no matter
what disaster you are standing in

A guide for easy mental stability for every day of your life.

ISBN - 9798622765827

Table of Contents

Table of Contents

Introduction

Even if you are in extreme physical and mental pain and are about to die, since you are the only life form off Planet Earth in the entire universe that could experience such events - you just have to learn how to enjoy it!

*This is the baseline for belief in being **Neutral or Better**. If you can read this, then that means you are alive and all complaints should stop there. The concept is simple: you need to be ALIVE to feel terrible. Being alive is above all. If "life" is required to feel terrible, then being ALIVE should be foremost in your thoughts.*

The next time you feel awful, terrible, or as if life is not worth living, you have to stop and grasp the concept that such emotions can only be possessed by a living being. You can't feel miserable if you are dead. To be human is to experience. Advanced humans are self-aware. Super advanced humans are aware of being self-aware. Self-aware humans know that human experience is unique in the entire universe. Self-aware humans understand that any discomfort in being alive is something that a rock or anything that is not alive just can't feel.

Life on Earth is abundant. Everywhere you look, there is life- it's hard to get away from it. Life off this planet is non-existence, as far as we know. Glancing up at the night sky what is visible is only a fraction of the universe. You are the only life form in this universe that can feel anything. So whenever life goes from bad to extreme worse, you just have to learn how to enjoy it. This concept is not that difficult. Appreciating being alive should be the baseline for happiness.

If you believe in heaven and are waiting to feel good after you die, well then – good luck with that. Waiting to feel good either after you die or waiting to feel happy for something or waiting to feel happy for another human's action is a complete and total waste of time. It is possible for any human to feel fantastic without the validation from any other human.

A human controls one of the universe's most amazing machines and of course, this machine is the human body. This fact alone needs to be celebrated on a daily basis. If you can grasp the concept that as a human machine operator, the world IS literately at your fingertips.

Inner Hippie

Try to channel your inner 1960's hippie. That persona is one of wonderment. Imagine a hippie who just smoked a Marijuana cigarette. Imagine that hippie holding up their hand and wiggling their fingers and speaking in a slow and amazed tone of voice, "Wow man, look what I can do with my fingers. Wow man, I can move my entire arm anyway I can think of. I can stand up and walk around the world if I wanted to." Humans should be as amazed with their body as that 1960's hippie is. With an understanding that control of a human body is a gift from some unknown power and the appreciation of this gift should dominate all thought.

A simpler concept is that being able to see your fingers wiggle constitutes two impossible actions. Moving your fingers in any capacity and being able to see your fingers move are two actions that are both impossible. If all your actions being a human are constituted as "impossible," your appreciation for whatever you do will slowly begin to emerge.

Baseline for human happiness should be a simple question: "Am I alive?" If the answer is yes, then everything should add to that concept, and nothing should ever subtract from it.

Rules: Becoming Neutral or Better

With the baseline of your human happiness defined, now it is time for a few details to help you achieve success with your day-to-day brain. (Don't tell anyone, but you have total control of your brain.)

Drama! Drama! Drama!

*Drama flows through humanity as oxygen permeates the planet. Drama seems to always be present and can be a terrible drain on the human psyche. Drama itself is unavoidable, but our absorption or reaction to any dramatic situations can be altered so that the impact from the experience is minimal, if not at all. The rules, mind games and techniques of **Neutral or Better** can suggest productive responses to mitigate the drama that we face in our day-to-day lives. With practice, all of these techniques will be ready for action when the need arises.*

*The best way to learn and implement **Neutral or Better** ideology is to first read the entire book from cover to cover. In these pages, you will find the techniques, rules, and mind games that could alter the view of a human existence. Being **Neutral or Better** begins with becoming self-aware with the eventual goal of going "manual human." Most humans run on autopilot 24 hours per day. Self aware humans should go manual when any type of drama begins to develop or at the height of major dramatic incident.*

Drama Can Be Entertainment

Each rule, technique or mind game can be used to create entertainment no matter how dire a situation can become. Humans still have to perform any duties that may be required, but turning drama into entertainment just may mitigate a negative experience.

As the concepts are revealed try to remember a personal situation where these concepts may have altered the outcome of a drama situation you may have experienced. If a recent personal drama situation is recognized while reading this book, then play a game of "what if?" Read the appropriate section several times (if necessary) and then imagine the same scenario being experienced in a different way. Imagine if the application of the rule, technique or mind game could have created a calmer environment or even entertainment rather than stress or discomfort.

*Imagine how just a slight change in your response might have reduced the impact on your mental state of affairs. Maybe the ideas of **Neutral or Better** could make dramatic encounters less emotionally taxing, and easier to live through. A key to this new way of thinking is recognizing that all of life can be a source of entertainment, even when it does not initially seem so.*

Being alive and interacting with other humans will always produce emotional and over the top experiences as with medical emergencies, drastic deadlines for work and even fighting in a shooting war. If you prepare your brain for drama by being self-aware, it is possible to keep emotionally calm and entertained. While this may seem unimaginable, every person can control how he or she thinks and feels. This is having the ability to apply this concept toward making life entertaining and enjoyable – no matter the barrier or hardships. This is not easy and will require continuing practice.

Each technique, rule or mind game can also be customized to your own personal style. Nothing suggested here is written in stone. This book is just a jumping-off point for you to start creating the best possible mental state for your life. The bottom line is that you are alive and that trumps any problem you may encounter. You can choose to live a satisfying and joyful life by the simple process of just becoming self-aware.

Welcome to Neutral or Better

Life is full of emotional roadblocks, pitfalls, and disasters, which mess with our psyche and disrupt our entire world. Family, friends, work, sickness, and even petty drama can suck the life right out of us. The psyche can sometimes seem to be a fragile Ming Vase just waiting to be knocked over to shatter into a thousand pieces. The gauntlet of life is a never-ending battle to keep our mental state from dropping into an abyss of depression or simply from just feeling lousy.

*The powerful, positive answers to this quagmire of emotions can be found in the rules, techniques and mind games of **Neutral or Better.** This book is a preemptive strike against all of the difficult things that may invade our mental world. These can be invasions of your* *conscious mind by other humans either by purposeful malice or just naiveté and their inability to aware of anything.*

*Your life could now possibly be set to cruise control. The key is keeping the mental state in a neutral or positive setting. This can be achieved when you simply start to maintain awareness of your own life and your surroundings. Being aware of your own emotions and the emotions of others can help deal with drama even before it happens. When prepared, all future dramas could only be an inconvenience, not a disaster and possibly a new source of entertainment. A few payments for "drama insurance" will pay off handsomely when drama inevitably make as occurrence in your life. **Neutral or Better** has you covered. Welcome to the club.*

Self-Awareness

*The most important aspect **Neutral or Better** is self-awareness. All concepts stem from being self-aware. Constant self-examination of your mental state during any given 24-hour period is the goal. What is the brain concentrating on? What outside influences are affecting the brain's thoughts? How is the brain handling the outside world's influence and intrusions? What concepts send the brain into a panic, or straight to a bout of severe depression?*

*To be **Neutral or Better** the humans needs to be constantly giving their mental state a status checkup. During normal human operation and happy times, being self-aware is very easy, but as the drama escalates self-awareness wanes. The emotions of the moment mask the ability to being self-aware, and this needs to be altered if **Neutral or Better** is desired. After much practice being self-aware at moments of extreme drama is possible. The time from drama and self-awareness is the gage on how in touch you are with your emotions. Normally, emotions take full control and add to mental anguish. As self-awareness becomes the focus, it will be possible that entertainment will replace mental anguish in all situations.*

*Being self-aware is the baseline for all of the remaining rules, techniques, and mind games of being **Neutral or Better**. It allows your natural state of being to remain on more neutral and controlled* *ground. Once self-awareness is a dominant concept, then life can change from the powerless reactive to the powerful pro-active, leading to a life of always being* **Neutral or Better**.

THE TWENTY-FIVE RULES
For Always Being Neutral or Better

1-Be self-aware

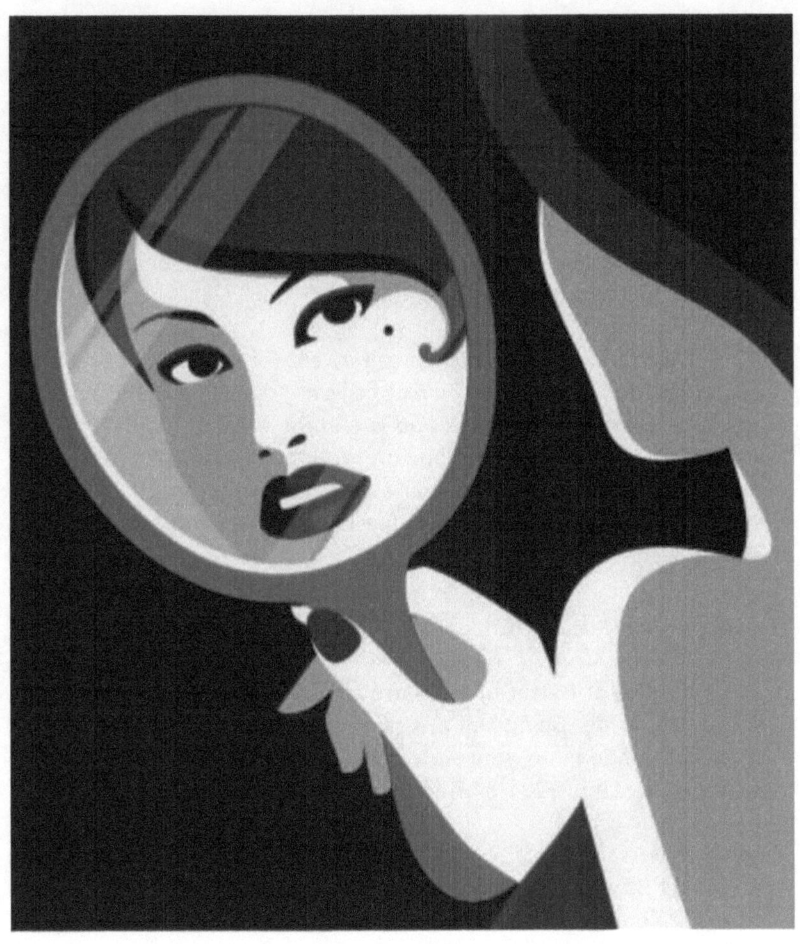

What is self-awareness? It is the simple state of consciousness that identifies that you are alive, that you see the world with your eyes, you hear the world with your ears, you feel the world with your fingers, and that you have complete control of your body and mind. It is realizing that you can do just about anything that you can imagine.

How Exactly do you FEEL?

Being self-aware is recognition of what your brain is doing at a particular moment in time. How do you feel? What emotions and bodily sensations are you experiencing? Do you feel good or bad? Do you feel happy or angry? Do you feel love or hate? In this state, thoughts are tangible so that you can observe and analyze your innermost workings. Being self-aware offers more control in life because even though emotions are very powerful – being self-aware allows you to balance the equation. The balance between emotions and rational thought needs to be equal.

To be **Neutral or Better** is to be self-aware for as much of any given 24-hour period as possible. Think of this as "reverse meditation." The goal is to calm your thoughts and live in the present moment. This is an exercise of self-reflection on your consciousness and sub-conscious. This is a state of hyper-awareness. When a human is in the state of **Neutral or Better**, then life is never lived on autopilot; it is always lived on manual.

Crystal Clear Observations

To be **Neutral or Better** humans are always aware of the "what, who, and why" of life. Being self-aware in any situation can offer crystal clear observations on your automatic reactions, and possibly create an instance of more successful decision-making.

Being self-aware will also supply information to you about how you are doing. Is your mind crying out for more information? The self-aware brain always knows that there is never an end to what can be learned. Being self-aware allows you to tune into to see how self-aware the people around you are. You can witness and determine if their lives are being ruled and controlled by the all-consuming emotional life.

2-Learn to be entertained by your MISERY

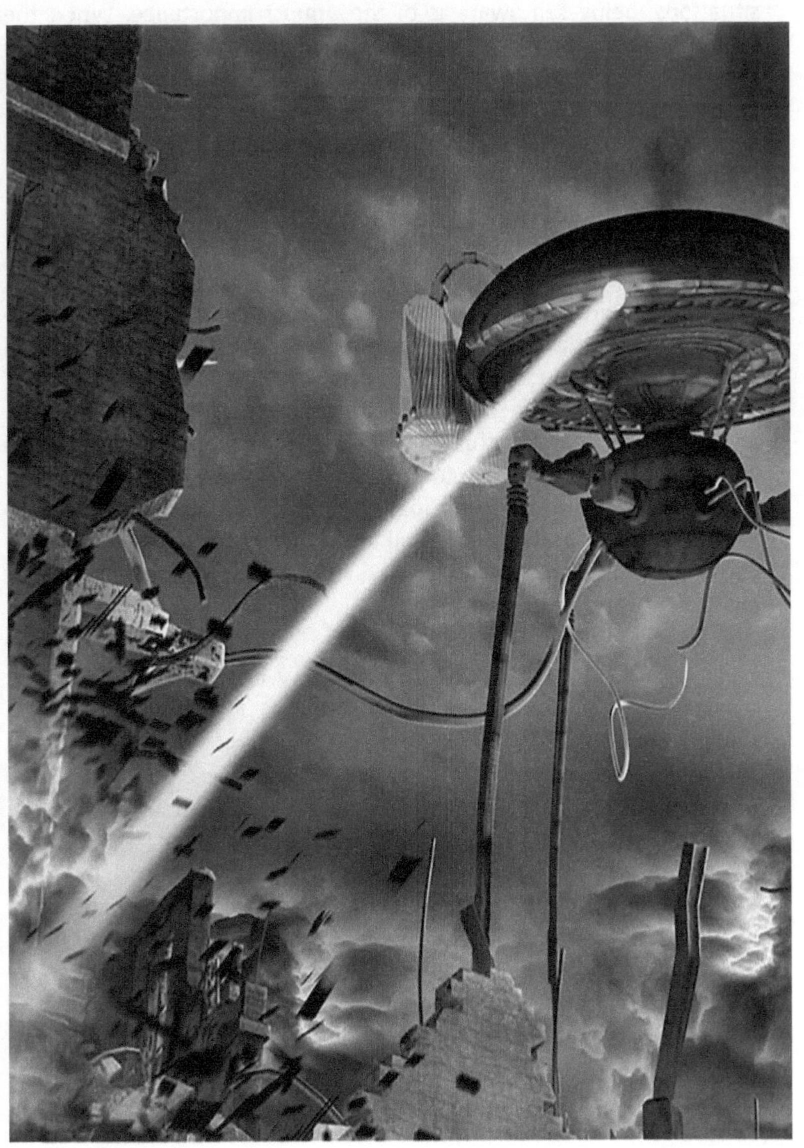

When a human is in a **Neutral or Better** state of mind this human never has a bad day. Even when the world is literally ending, life is entertaining if the correct frame of mind is achieved. In dramatic situations, being self-aware is of the utmost importance. When the drama is small, being self-aware is very easy. When the drama is severe, being self-aware is much more difficult. In the moment of true desperation emotions may become overwhelming. To be prepared for the big dramas in life, practice self-awareness during the small moments.

The Easiest Place to Practice

The good moments in life are the easiest places to practice self-awareness. The next time you have a great success or you are being entertained by friends and family, or you're just having a great day, take a step back and survey the scene. Why is this moment so enjoyable? What makes this slice of life so pleasurable? Writing down your observations may help to truly understand why you feel so good. Knowing what causes a great feeling is important. When the brain is happy, so is the body. And it's all about the body in the long run. If you know what can lead to happiness, it is easier to recreate or seek it out in the future.

Happy Brain Happy Body

There is one truth that trumps all others. This is also from a cliché that has permeated humanity for years – "find your bliss." So, what is up with finding bliss? It is really quite simple: when a person finds his or her bliss—whether it is religion, a relationship, a job, a hobby, or something else—the brain goes into a state of extreme happiness. When the brain is happy, the body has a good chance of operating at its highest efficiency. A body that is working well might live longer, and that's really all that matters. It doesn't matter what you believe in, or who, or what; finding anything that makes the brain happy will increase the longevity of the body, and that's the bottom line.

Standing over your newborn baby in the hospital may seem like the most serious moment in anyone's life, but what if the entire moment could be as entertaining as it is serious? Can people be entertained by disaster? Can we be entertained while risking our life trying to save the lives of hundreds of other humans?

The theory is that the more entertained a person is in the face of life circumstances (good or bad), the more efficiently they can operate. Instead of being nervous and apprehensive at a job interview, being entertained by the moment can allow for confidence and calm operation, allowing you to make the best possible impression on the recruiter. If a police officer is entertained by a dramatic situation, he may not react poorly and shoot when it isn't needed. Find a way to interpret a bad situation in a positive or neutral way through looking at it as entertainment or a storyline.

Pre-Surgery Entertainment

Humans make decisions every day regarding hundreds of scenarios. Making a conscious decision to be entertained regarding an upcoming situation may indeed create a more positive outcome. The body follows the brain. The body follows the brain's clues. If before any type of surgery, the brain is entertained days, hours and minutes before going under the knife, the body will respond in kind.

(Author's Note: I recently had hip replacement surgery. Hip replacement is a common occurrence but still a major surgery. I started weeks before preparing my body and my mind for the event. I ate the recommended foods, vitamins and performed the required exercises. I also prepared my mind by initiating an entertainment protocol. I decided to be completely entertained by the upcoming surgery and I held that thought until I was knocked completely out in the operating room.

My mental preparation accomplished two things: my mind and body were ready for the surgery and responded well to the operation and I had absolute no worries about what was coming. Why would you be worried about something that would be entertaining? That's the key to this mind game. Replacing fear of the unknown to a certainty of entertainment.

I'm seven weeks removed from surgery and my results are 120% positive.)

Real Disasters

In a true disastrous situation as in a hurricane, tsunami, brush fire, earthquake or even in a pandemic, the human brain that is entertained will function at a much higher level of efficiency.

How can a human brain be entertained when the world all around is falling apart?   How can disaster become entertainment? Being entertained by a disaster is a multi-step process which begins by looking at the past years of your life.   The past years need to be examined and then realized that being alive is just an impossibility and the excitement and drama, good and bad, just doesn't exist anywhere else in the universe. Once these past years are appreciated to a point where gratitude is introduced, the present day disaster becomes what it should be: just another adventure in this fabulous thing called life.

Survival – The Most Important Directive

The human brain provides each human operator with many directives for the care and feeding of each human being. The most important directive present in the conscious and subconscioure is of course survival of the human machine. Every action taken by a human is somehow related to survival. Every actions, thought, word or deed of any human is related to the survival of that human. The subconscious is responsible for most of technical operation of the human body including breathing. The conscious is responsible to find food, water and shelter. All these operations keep the body alive.

Survival: Pleasure and Pain

Everything the human mind is consciously thinking of is designed for the continuing survival the human machine. Having fun, sex, eating, going to the movies, attending school and traveling on vacation are all designed to keep the brain happy and when the brain is happy it is easier to survive. When something happens that could make survival more difficult, then the mind begins to worry and that should only be a triggering action not a way of life.

Devise The Perfect Plan!

 When an earthquake, flood, brushfire, pandemic, medical condition or unemployment take place then these events should trigger a response action. The response action should involve a plan and this plan should be written down. The plan may require days or even weeks to compile, but once the plan is in place the mental state of the human should go back to the neutral state. Once the plan has been determined then there is no reason to spend additional time worrying. Look at the plan as a security blanket or any devise that offers a soothing feeling. The human brain functions much better when the mental state is closer to neutral. Being Neutral or Better may take some practice, but all humans need to make this state mind their goal.

Entertained by Misery

Becoming self aware and being able to be entertained by disasters, big and small, will alert any human to new way of the enjoyment of being alive. Humans need to realize that life is this impossible gift that should be enjoyed no matter what is happening. When the aliens do invade, humanity will be much better equipped to fight off the invasion if we are entertained rather then being scared to death.

3-Take nothing personally especially when it is

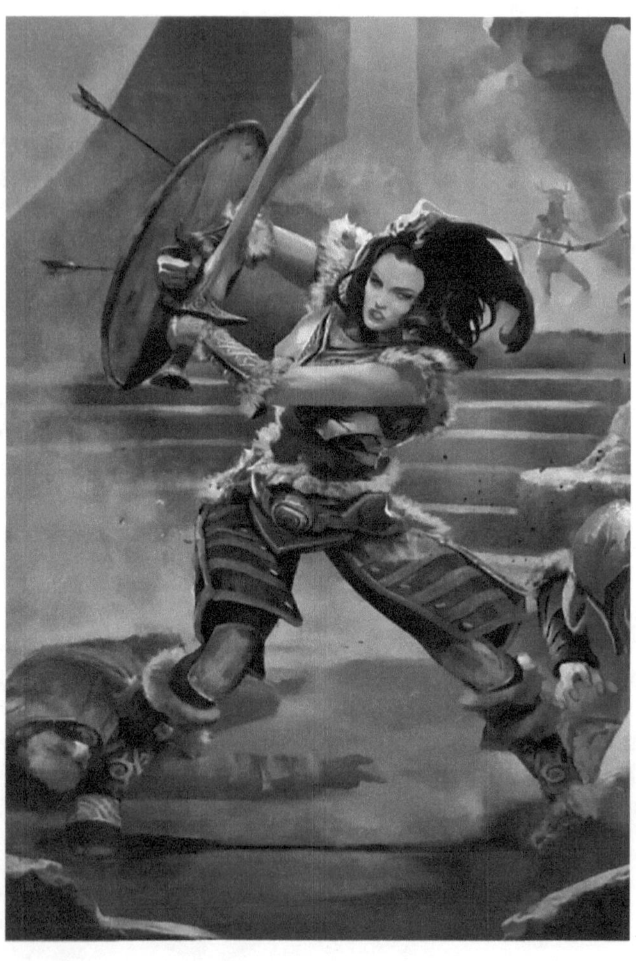

This is just as the age-old cliché says: "sticks and stones can break my bones, but words will never hurt me."

In day-to-day life the following questions will arise more often than not: What did they really mean when they said that? Was there a hidden message? Were they trying to insult me? In the world of **Neutral or Better** who cares about any of this? Let it go. There is zero benefit to worrying or creating strife before it even happens. You control your brain, so even if their intentions were derogatory, why give them the satisfaction of negative impact on your life?

One way to deal with the uncertainty behind the actions of others is to always assume remarks are directed at your true self. Assume he or she has insulted your core existence. Once you do this, you can convince yourself that those remarks are the worst possible insults you could ever experience. And that is it; they are just words. You didn't get physically hurt. They didn't destroy your being. They don't have that power. So, just have a laugh and move on! Remember, words are only words, and only you have to power to change the way you feel.

Search for Value in Remarks

Now, in some cases, you may want to evaluate the remarks. They may have value, and maybe you can learn something from them, or grow from the experience. This needs to be done when separated from the emotional moment at a later date or time. Examples of remarks that should be evaluated are criticism from an employer or medical advice from a doctor or lawyer. Anything said in such cases should certainly be evaluated.

Some people go "defensive" at a moment's notice no matter what is said to them. When a human is in a **Neutral or Better** state of mind, they are allowed 10 seconds to feel that "emotional dagger," and then rational thought must take over. The more you internally contemplate the remark the more you can truly evaluate it. After a deep breath, the response should always be, 'that's a good point." Do not dismiss any criticism or suggestion at first light, evaluate all and accept the good and discard the meaningless.

As a last note, if someone aims to defame or accuses you of a crime that you didn't commit, please contact a lawyer. That becomes a more serious matter and a different situation entirely.

4-Remove emotionally linked words from your vocabulary

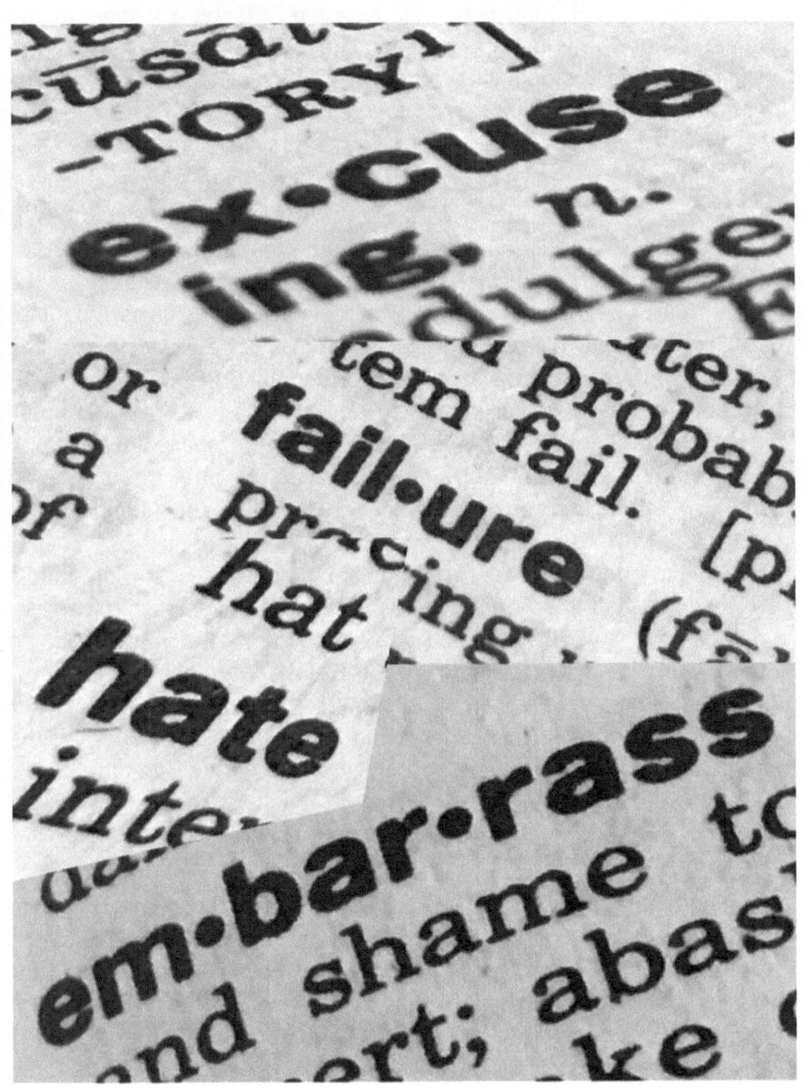

Emotions are tied to words, and words are tied to emotions. There are many trigger words that can bring on negative emotions that alter your experiences in life. To maintain a calm and comfortable state of mind, there are many words that should be deleted from your vocabulary, both internally and externally. If words that trigger negative emotions do not exist in your world, then you can more easily maintain a stable and calm state of being. This rule can also be considered a "Mind Game" with yourself.

Offended – The Word Does Not Exist

There are also words that exist which are commonly used as insults. These can be directed toward your way of life, your religion, or the essence of your being. You may realize that the insult is meant to cause emotional distress because of the link between words and emotions. If, for instance, the word "offended" does not exist in your vocabulary, then you can never truly be offended. Consciously break the link between the negative word(s) and the impact they have on your emotions. As with any new concept, this may require some practice, effort, and concentrated energy to fully receive the benefit.

The next time you feel offended by someone or something, remember that the word "offended" doesn't have to hold any real meaning for you. This is just a simple mind game that you can play to trick your brain into staying in a neutral state. You get to control how you feel when you are aware of how some words can affect your brain. Take control of your mind and consciousness; you've had the ability since before you were born. All you need to do is tap into it.

Embarrassed – The Word Does Not Exist

Feeling embarrassed may prevent you from experiencing all that you can because it can cause you to close yourself off. Eliminating "embarrassment" (and related words) from your vocabulary can thus help mitigate the reactive mental state, which is really just fear of what other people think. Who cares what they think about you? Really, all that matters are what you think about yourself, and if you are aware, other people's thoughts don't have to impact you.

Eliminating this concept may even open up an entirely new world for you to explore and enjoy.

Eliminating the word "segreto" from your vocabulary is self-explanatory. You need to change your belief system so that there are no regrets, only life. Regret may cause you to fall into depression when, in actuality, it is just an opportunity to learn from past experiences. Eliminate this, and instead of dwelling on the past, you can move forward to your future.

The Word – EXCUSE Does Not Exist

There should never be any excuses for something that goes wrong. Eliminate "excuse" from your vocabulary so that you can live in the present moment and learn from mistakes. Make sure that any situation, whether good or bad, doesn't come down to making an excuse. Own your story and your life. Instead of coming up with excuses, plan ahead! Plan for deadlines, try to figure out what could go wrong, and prepare for it. If you are ready for the worst-case scenario, you will not be fazed if something actually does go wrong. Even when it seems as though the world has turned against you, never give an excuse; just say, "It will be okay. Now I know, and it won't happen again."

Replace HATE with Indifference

"Hate" is such a powerful word, and can even result in the slaughter of millions of people. On a personal level, hate requires an enormous amount of energy. Allocate your energy to positive emotions and words. By eliminating "hate," you eliminate the ability to hate or be hated. Now, love also requires energy, but there will be a positive impact on life by focusing excess energy on love. Take the energy that was spent on hate and redirect it to something positive. If disliking something is really that important, then the trick is to not hate, but to be "indifferent." Being indifferent is so much more powerful and easier than hating. Hate is a total waste of your energy! Indifference is much closer to a neutral state of being. Save your energy, move all hated things or people into a non-existent column in your life. Delete "hatred" from your vocabulary!

Fear of Failure

Fear of failure and rejection are ever present for most people, and these emotions are often related to the completion of a task. It is important to remember that most things can be done more than once, so there is no need to fear failure on the first attempt. When a **Neutral or Better** state of mind is in progress there are endless future possibilities, and one of those will eventually be successful. "Failure" is a word and concept that should not be recognized; it is just an opportunity to try something again and do better next time. A single non-successful attempt at anything is only one attempt and must be embraced as only one attempt. The remaining hundred to one thousand attempts are the key to success. You must be self-aware enough to stay calm amidst your fear so that you can focus on doing your best, and your future successes.

5-Realize that no one owes you anything

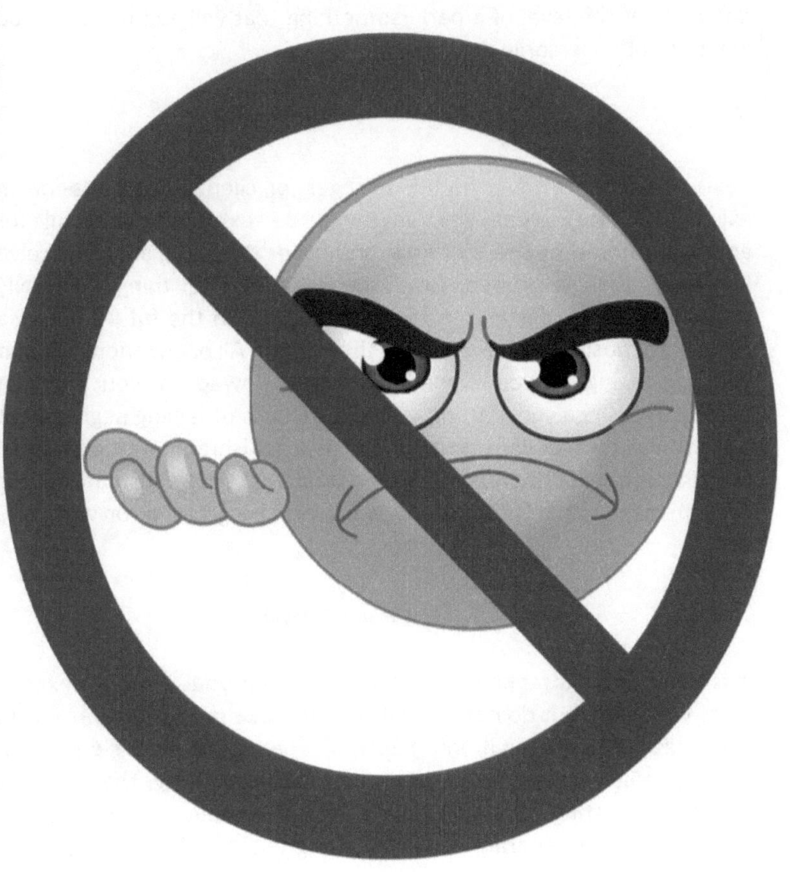

How many times have you heard of someone longing for validation from a parent, loved one, friend or fan? When a mind is Neutral or Better this is a waste of energy! What could possibly be accomplished by waiting for somebody else to validate you? Of course, this works for a job situation, but not for day-to-day relationships. Waiting for an emotional handoff from someone else is a waste of energy and time. If you absolutely will die without validation, then place this emotional apple pie at the level of a perk (something that will add to your good life, but not necessarily define it).

Gratitude is Powerful

Realize that no relative, friend, stranger, or client (unless it's for an existing invoice) owes you anything. Be extremely grateful for anything offered by these groups, and never think you should receive any more than is offered. Gratitude is a powerful thing. Generally showing that you are grateful will benefit you in the future because people get positive reactions from that action. Also, any thoughts that you are being denied something that is owed to you are just destructive. Once you start down the dark path of feeling neglected, it will forever control your destiny. This is a selfish and entitled way of thinking about life. It ends up being a waste of energy. Instead, always do your best, work for what you want, and be grateful for what you get.

Disappointment

It is okay to be disappointed, especially when you don't get exactly what you want, but do not let that thought take over and control you. The rules say that even if only a 10th of what is expected is delivered, take it, smile and move on. When you expect nothing, then there is never any lasting disappointment. When people do deliver, the unexpected can generate a particularly great day. The concept that takes self-awareness to another level is always re-directing thoughts from negative to positive. Be aware of any negative thoughts and immediately create a positive thought to counter the negative. This will take practice but remembering to this do this exercise will keep the mind **Neutral or Better.**

Humans should be their own greatest fan. Constantly offering validation and self-care is a very easy exercise to improve mental health. Humans enjoys something that is a singular experience in the entire universe and that is being alive. Learn to enjoy it, always!

6-Own the emotions in your life then forget the details

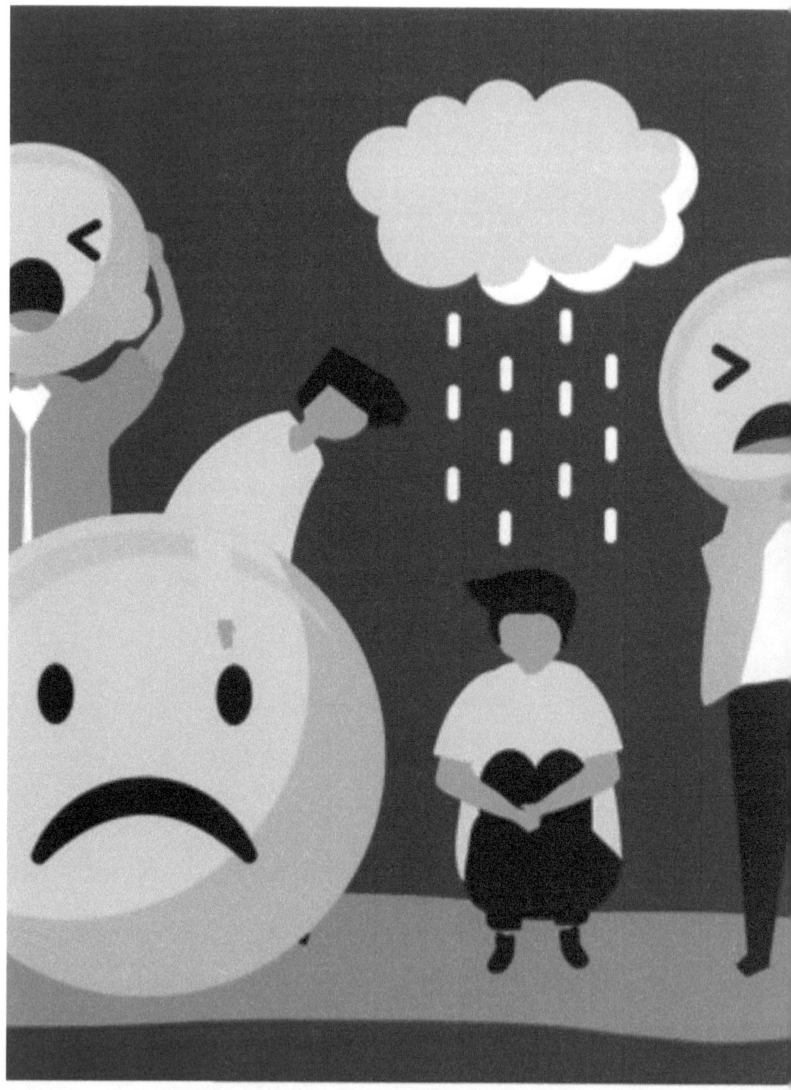

No Blame after Twenty-Five

There is a joke that essentially says: "a child can't blame his or her parents for any lack of training, or an overall horrible existence, once the child turns 25." If anyone could be blamed for creating a dysfunctional person, it could certainly be the parents; but blaming the parents for anything is just a waste of energy. To be **Neutral or Better**, a human never blames his or her parent(s) for anything. Instead, they simply take what has been offered to them and build up their life from there. From parents physically doing harm to providing the best of everything, once a child leaves the nest, its their life. You need to own the emotions linked to your childhood but forget the petty details. You can always do better in the future. Whatever you didn't get, go get it yourself now.

Determine What is Missing and Learn It

Blaming someone for things that they did or didn't do is basically an exercise in just slamming your own head against a wall. This accomplishes nothing but self-inflicted wounds. If you are alive, be thankful, and use the most amazing machine in the universe to get what you want: your brain and body. You can do virtually anything! If your parents did not teach you certain skills, then go learn those skills from someone else. If your parents offered nothing but bad advice, then find a source of true enlightenment.

Negative Role Models

There are such things as "negative role models" who serve as models for what not to do in life. If parents are determined to have been negative role-models, then being aware of this fact is the first step into a much wider world of existence. Knowing what is a negative can be helpful be very helpful as there is now a template on what is not helpful. Failure is the best teacher.

Letting Go of the Past

Being Neutral or Better allows the of letting go of all past injustices, failures, bad relationships and betrayals. Every human truly lives between the ears and that space needs to be made into the most enjoyable space in the universe.

The Best They Could Do

If a marriage ended in a terrible divorce, that is now in the past. Realizing that the two humans in that failed marriage did the best that was possible and now it is time to move on. Whatever evil and terrible things happened to any human in the past, to create a Neutral or Better state of mind these humans have to own the emotions, learn from the experience then move past the details. Focus on what can learned from the experience. Humans can always choose to look at a negative experience with a positive outlook. This leads to a positive overall view of life. Failure is the absolute best teacher.

Own The Emotions

When it comes to the memory of the event itself, feelings, emotions, and reactions are more important than the details. Hanging on to something specific (especially that happened multiple years ago) is a waste of energy, and can only be self-destructive. Just realize that the past can be viewed, and reviewed, and analyzed, but never changed. Don't dwell on the details of a negative past event. Use your energy to create a positive future.

7-Always anticipate that 100 attempts will be required to achieve anything of importance

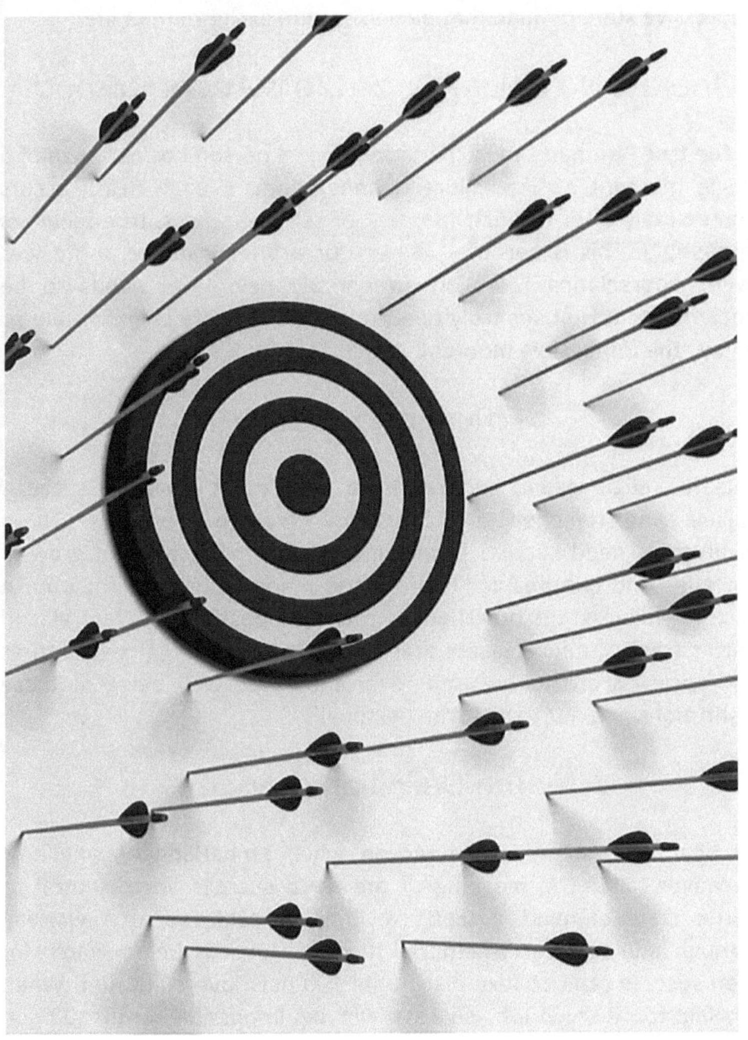

Two of the enemies of being **Neutral or Better** are rejection and failure. These things are common occurrences in anyone's life. School, dating, jobs, sports, business, and everything else can be soaked with rejection and failure. There is no escape from either, but there is a method that can squash the negative emotions that they bring up. What does enabling failure and rejection offer? They only offer a depressive state of mind that diminishes the excitement of life.

There is No Failure Once Life is Accomplished

In the true "Human Zen" experience, once a person has partaken of a single moment of life, failure is nonexistent. Even if death occurs immediately after the first moment of self-awareness, true failure is impossible. This is because, if even for a brief instance, a life was lived. Appreciating "life" on an entirely new level needs to be implemented. Humans truly need to realize that life is impossible so enjoy **"the impossible moment"** that is life!

Failure and Society

Society, religions and cultures have a different views of success. Failure and rejection are constantly deemed worthless. These institutions need success from humans as a mechanism of growth. Societies and cultures can't afford too many failures so they make sure all failures are punished as much as possible. A Neutral and Better state of mind realizes that statements from religions, cultures and societies are to be used to promote the well being of these institutions and not to be taken personally.

Alter The Definition of Success

To deal with failure and rejection when embarking on any new endeavor, alter the meaning of the word success. In a Neutral or Better state of mind, **success** can only be achieved after working through one hundred attempts. If a new lover is being search for then success can not take place until 100 new lovers are met. When looking for a new job, success will be impossible until 100 job interviews have taken place. When looking for new place to live, the perfect accommodation will not be accepted until 100 hones or apartments are inspected.

The Mind Game of Success

This is a powerful way of thinking, no matter how difficult your journey might seem to be. As you work towards the 100th attempt, something unexpected will happen. Usually, around 20 or 30 attempts, you will be directed to something, or you will meet someone you never even thought about, that will be a direct key to your future success. If you do make 100 attempts at something and have no success, then yes move on to something else.

8-Men 30 seconds
Women 5 minutes

Life is very short! When a human brain is in a **Neutral or Better** state it realizes and makes sure the highest percentage of this short life is experienced with a positive attitude. Depression is a natural emotion that settles into the brain when: life either removes something or someone from our world, fear of the unknown creeps in, something expected is not fulfilled, a favorite sports team loses the big game, or we experience countless other unwanted losses. The list of human depression activators is endless. Neutral or Better minds knows immediately when depression sets in. Super self aware humans can even see depression approaching.

Embrace Depression

The rules regarding depression are simple: embrace the feeling of the depression, go as deep as possible into the depression, bring on the self-pity, create a mental scenario that leads to the worst possible feeling and worst mental anguish you can image. Once you have hit rock bottom and you can't go any deeper, take a step back and start laughing. After laughing, you may return to the deep depression state of mind or not. This exercise can demonstrate the power of the amazing brain. It shows that changing your depression can truly only be a laugh away.

Thirty Seconds for Men

A **Neutral or Better** state of mind knows that this pity party is only allowed for thirty seconds (women are allowed five minutes), and then you have to get to work. In reality, life's depressions can be devastating. Our brains sometime can't handle what life throws at us, or they cannot "get around" a devastating loss. The number one rule to remember is that "life is short." People need to grieve when presented with all sorts of emotional events. The key is to not let the depression endure longer than it has to. When a Neutral or Better state of mind exists this mind is self aware of the depression. There is no doubt. No one needs to ask "Are you dressed?" Self aware humans are constantly gauging how depressed they are and how much longer they will need to feel "bad." This is very important: A **Neutral or Better** mind controls when the depression will end.

Scare Yourself Silly

An easy way to lessen the effects of depression is to challenge yourself to a task in which you been avoiding all your life. This type of action may indeed change your life forever and turn your depression into a positive. So, depression has sent in, you feel awful. You really can't feel any worse, so why not try something that has always scared you? At this point, we have already determined that your feelings have bottomed out; there is no way to feel worse. Just go for it! During this journey of depression, it is your duty to yourself to attempt something that you have avoided all your life. People avoid trying all sorts of things because of fear of rejection or failure. This is the perfect time to try.

Going Past Normal

If you already feel as low as possible, you have nothing to lose in the attempt of something new. Not only will this attempt at something new offer you the possibility of a small triumph, but also, just maybe, it will lessen your depression. When you find yourself in hell, you have two choices: stay in hell, or figure out a way to climb back to normal life. The benefit in climbing back to normal is that during your journey, you will learn things that might enable you to go past normal for a new and better existence.

Facing Your Fears

Author's note: Before I starting writing this book I fell into a deep depression over a failed relationship. The depression was mind boggling. Later, I determined the depression was caused by just completing feeling sorry for myself due to the lost of what I considered the most important relationship of my life (It only lasted seven weeks from start to finish). Anyway, during the depression I had to get my mind off what I was going through. I recently learned how to surf and was competent in waves no more than four feet high. I needed a distraction from the depression I was going through so I decided to go surfing in waves close to eight feet high. For two hours I didn't catch many waves, but I completely forgot about my depression. For two hours all I could think about was staying alive. Towards the end of the surf session I was driven so deep by a wipe-out that I was forced underwater for what seemed like an eternity. After that wave, I crawled out of the water and realized I had beaten my depression due to the intensity of the activity. My depression returned when I arrived back home, but I knew then my condition was not permanent and I would recover. When I finally did emerge from the black hole of my depression I asked why I had done this to myself. I kept asking more questions and I finally asked "why does any human do anything?" Out of my depression I created a complete philosophy that answers all my question about humanity and this book is just a sliver of what I think II have discovered. Bottom line, use your next depression to scare the hell out of yourself and don't be surprised about what you'll discover about things you never even knew existed.

Not a Cure for Clinical Depression

Neutral or Better rules probably will not work with clinical depression, but any opportunity to avoid drugs should always be considered. It may seem easier to languish in a depressed state on a doctor's prescription then to face the ugly truth that may lie deep in the subconscious.

There are approximately 50,000 suicides per year in The United States. These are humans where the pain of living has overwhelmed the survival directives that is the main subroutine of the human operating system. This type of brain has been damaged from birth or has be inflicted with an event either biological or social. This type of human brain has been unable to save. The scoreboard doesn't lie: Drugs/Counseling Zero * Damaged Brains 50,000.

The next level of depression are humans who have been on anti depressants for more than two years. This group numbers about twenty- five million in the US. Neutral or Better rules may offer a very small percentage of this group some insight on how to move away from drugs and regain control of their lives. The next group, the rest od humanity, is where Neutral and Better rules will be most effective.

9-Take 100% of the responsibility for everything in your life

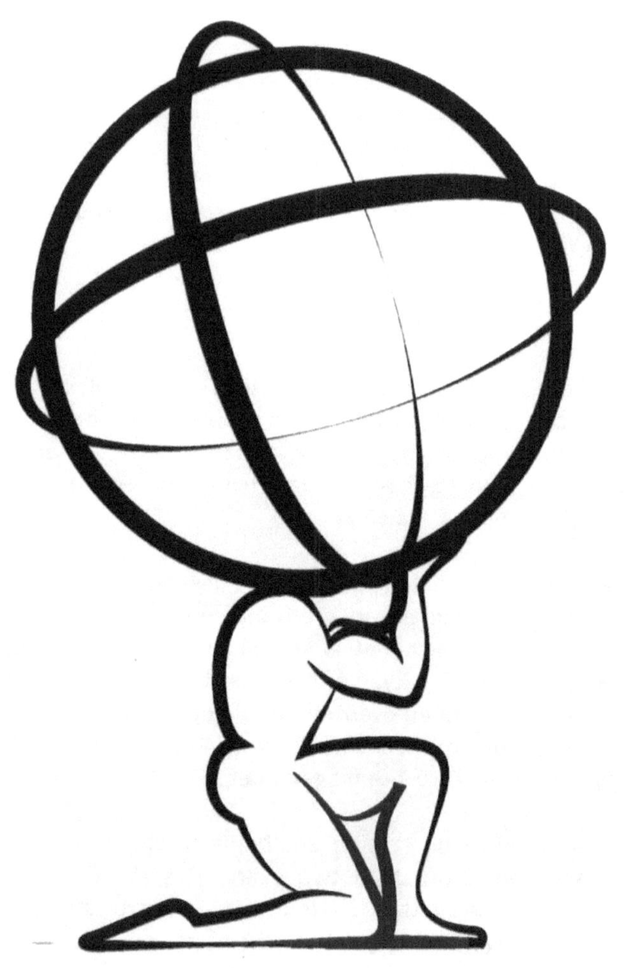

The "Blame Pie" does not exist in the world of being Neutral or Better. There is no percentage of blame divided up between any others besides yourself. To be a truly Neutral or Better human, one should accept 100% of the responsibility for everything that occurs in life. This is a mind game so that your brain isn't wasting time or energy trying to blame anyone else. **Just take responsibility for everything in your life even for events and circumstances you have or had no control over.**

Don't Give Up Any Power

Assigning blame equals a loss of power, and your power should never be given up to anyone. When blame is directed at others, a solid weakness is revealed.

Take Control of Life

A Neutral or Better state of mind never is allowed to wallow in the glow of blaming someone else. Taking 100% responsibility will lead to better circumstances in the future. When all of the responsibility is embraced, then all the moving parts—even the ones where you have no influence—must also be embraced. When every single moving part in life is accounted for, then the true work can begin. Here are some simple explanations: 1) If the dog has been eating your homework, give the dog away. 2) If traffic prevents you from being on time, move closer to work 3) If parking tickets are a problem, sell your car 4) If you can't win a poker, stop gambling 5) If you don't have any friends, learn how to find and make friends 6) If you want a girlfriend, learn how to be girlfriend material 8) And so on.

Influence The Outcome

Always build redundancies into all your plans. Think about the parties you can't control and try to figure out how to influence the outcome to suit you. Once you realize that all situations can be affected by pre-thought, you can truly take 100% on the responsibility, and thus, 100% of the credit! The easiest way to remain calm and enjoy life is to spend extra time on everything (maybe even twice the time). This is a simple rule that offers spectacular results.

10-Nothing is Unfair

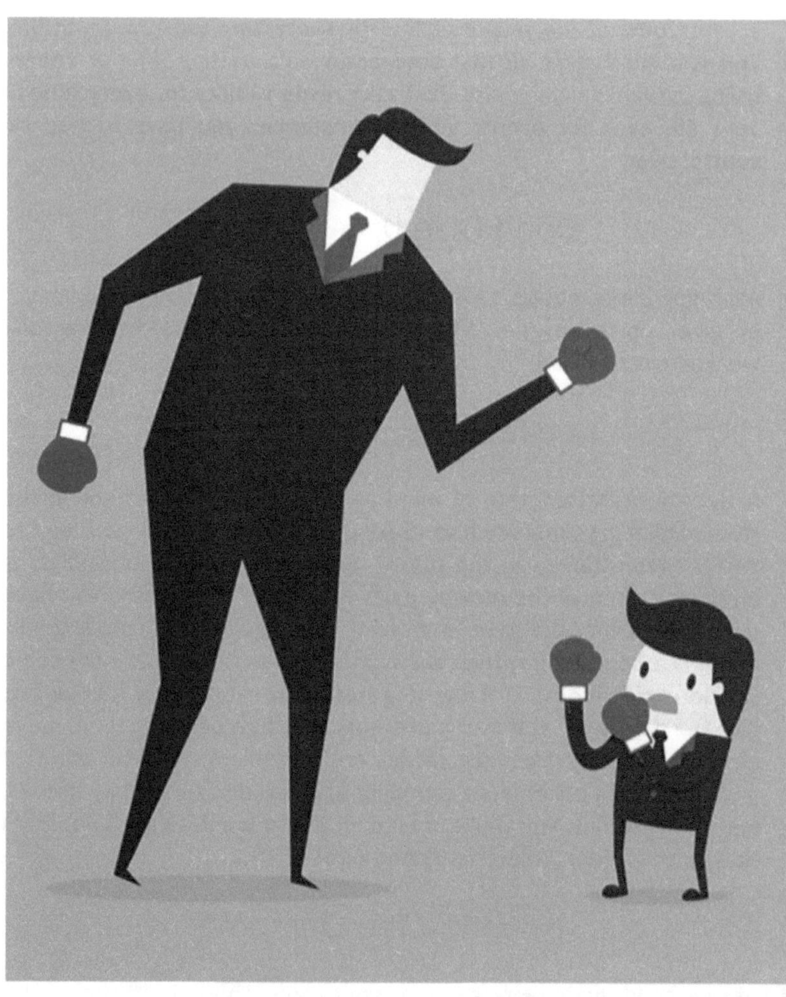

Being Neutral or Better offers the ability to survey life constantly and to always remember that being alive trumps everything. When someone utters the phrase "life is unfair," they fail to recognize that having life in the first place obliterates any notion of unfairness. Being alive is ridiculously amazing! Being alive is beyond comprehension.

Life is a Gift from Beyond

Being alive is a gift from somewhere, from someone, from something, and every second should be cherished. Now, tell me again...what exactly is unfair about life?

Information – People - Situation

Once the concept of "being alive" is held as the most important concept of all, then you can tackle any other problem you might have. When any situation appears to have a degree of unfairness, immediately remember that the concept does not exist. Situations are not unfair; maybe you don't have the correct information, do not know the correct people, or are truly in the wrong situation for you at the moment.

Take Complete Control

To determine what exactly is happening, take a step back from your emotions and review the entire situation. What is not happening the way you expected? All decisions made by others (which concern your life) involve many factors. If you are not receiving the credit, work, respect, et cetera, that you think you should, why is that? It is not because life is unfair; maybe life just demands you do some more work, work harder, or even heaven forbid, remove yourself from the situation. If you have to quit a job, get a divorce, or move to another part of the country to be successful – then do it!

Unfair Equals Hopeless

Never give up any power by arbitrarily stating that things are unfair. When things are unfair there is no recourse. Situations with no recourse are hopeless and being Neutral or Better never allows any situation to be hopeless. Always look to change your live for the better, and take action!

11-Learn how to step back from your emotions and judge all situations on other criteria

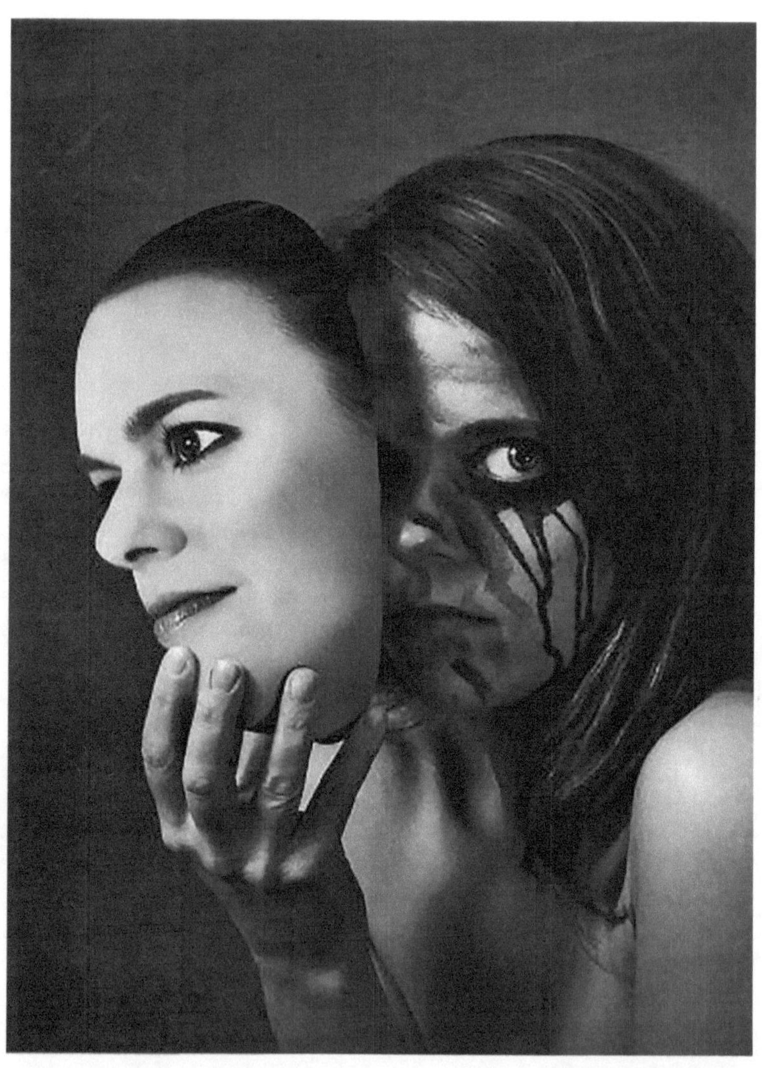

Being Neutral or Better begins and ends with self-awareness, so realizing which emotions are driving your actions is very important. When any type of drama appears (especially unexpectedly), certain emotions seize your brain and can dictate how you act or react. All types of major drama that involve accidents and injuries immediately heighten every human emotion, and the pertinent, survival ones are then put into play. The holy grail of self-awareness is being able to step away from your emotions in a major bodily injury.

Intense Drama Requires Focused Action

Imagine being a pedestrian in a hit-and-run accident late at night. You are alone and in extreme pain because your femur is now poking through your pant leg. How would you react, and how would you feel? The advanced self aware human would only allow for a few seconds of extreme panic and fear to consume their conscious mind, before calming down and taking serious action. The thought that "yes, you're going to die" should replace the fear of dying as quickly as possible. Once death has been determined as a possibility (especially if you just sit there and wait for it to happen), then there is nothing else to lose. It is time to get to work! Being completely self aware would know that the most important survival action would be to get off the road somehow. Being hit by another car is the worst possible next case scenario. Instead of crying out in pain and hoping someone hears you, take action and get yourself out the way of any oncoming cars. Once you've reached the shoulder, you can yell for help, and even pass out, if needed. Being self-aware at critical life or death moments is the ultimate way to be entertained, even if it seems difficult or impossible in the moment.

Go to The Worst Case Scenario

The preceding example is a worst-case scenario, but the practicality of accepting your fate can be done in any case. It can be the most calming action a fragile brain can perform in times of need. When you instantly accept the worst case result, then fear will not be a factor in your recovery. "Remain calm" is the credo for these sorts of situations, but "how can you remain calm if you are worried about the worst that can happen?" you may ask. The key is to accept that the worst can (and possibly will) happen and that there is nothing that can change that fact. So, do what you can to prevent it, get to work and impact the outcome.

Worrying about something is the worst possible mental state to be in. Instead, bypass "what could happen" and accept "it has already happened" or "it will happen."

Impending Disaster at 70 MPH

Author's note: Here's a personal experience where I accepted my fate and was saved by that action.

While I was driving at seventy miles per hour on an LA freeway, a multi-car wreck began in the lanes off to my right. Due to the proximity of the cars involved I immediately just assumed that I would be part of the collision. Several cars had decided to crash into each other and their swirling out of control mass of mangled auto parts was spinning directly for the pace in front of my car. As I witnessed this real time disaster I accepted the fact I too would soon be engulfed in this conflagration. By doing so my mind was free to work out a solution.

Free the Mind

Since I had accepted my fate my mind raced with the possible outcome. How much damage would this accident inflict on my body? I knew for sure my tiny sport cars would soon be reduced to just pieces metal clutter. I imagined being spun into this wreck with other vehicles landing on top of me. All this of course is happening in a blink of an eye, which demonstrates just how fast the human brain can work. After my brain calculated the outcome of this impending doom, the idea of escape flash before me. Without wasting another micro second I stomped on the gas pedal and moved to the next lane accelerating from 70 to almost 100 mph. As I passed the collision I was instantly pelted with disembodied parts from the four vehicles who now had created a loud smoking screeching mess of tangled metal.

Clear Thinking and Luck

Several factors contributed to my thrilling escape. The fact that no one was in the lane next to me and that I was able to accelerate out of trouble helped considerably. As I checked my read view mirror all I could see were flames and black deadly smoke.

I avoided the worst-case scenario by taking action through acceptance and a calm state of self-awareness. The brain really can only do one thing at a time well; it cannot worry and be active simultaneously. Let your brain do what it can: accept your fate, and then get to work!

Walking Away - Best Policy

Sometimes walking away is the best policy—Neutral or Better minds never take part in a fight. Being self-aware will always prevent this. Instead of verbally sparring with someone as they sink into a self-destructive state of mind, try to reason with the other person. Try to get the core reason for the confrontation. If the combative opponent refuses to listen to reason and continues the fight, then it is best to just walk away and not participate. If the fighter just will not let it go, continue to avoid engagement, and keep walking away. You do not need to give them the fight that they are looking for because you need to stay Neutral or Better. Never choose to engage.

12-Unless someone slams a two by four against your head, no one should control the way you feel

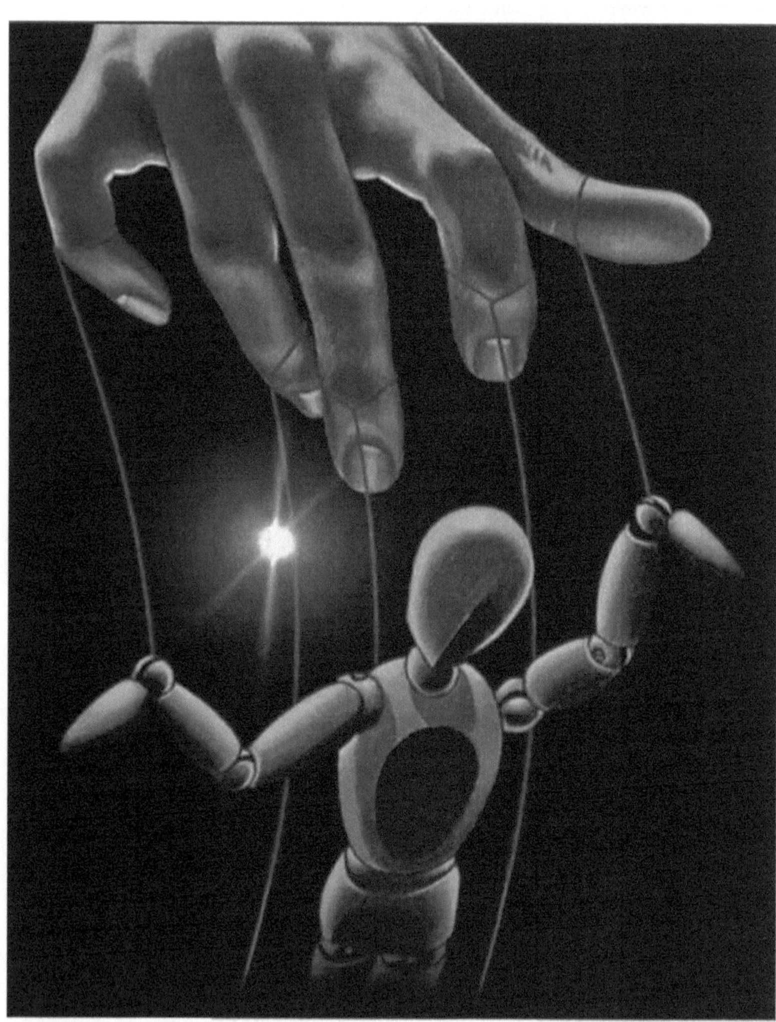

Imagine living your day-to-day life with a slightly different set of rules. The new rules may seem very strange, but let it be; this is a very fun exercise.

Everyone Carries a 2 x4

 In this make-believe world, everyone you meet, talk to, or interact with will be carrying a 2" x 4" wood board on their shoulder. Usually, this would only happen if you are friends with a carpenter who's framing a new home, but in this make-believe world, everyone has a 2 x 4. Now imagine that everyone you interact with slams that 2 x 4 against your head if you disagree with them, and every time you feel pain and discomfort. There is no way not to feel pain. The physical contact itself must generate pain because the contact stimulates the nerves in the body, and sends signals to the brain, and the reaction creates an uncomfortable sensation. The key to see this situation is that a 2 x 4 is making physical contact with you. Physical contact is the only way you will really feel pain.

Now, let's go back to the real world. How many people in your life carry 2 x 4s? How many are swinging that 2 x 4 at your head? How many are making contact with your head with a piece of wood? How often do you bleed from said blow? A wild guess is "never."

No Physical Contact

If there is no physical contact, then how can anyone affect the way you feel? Many people in your day-to-day life will try to affect your brain's reactions by saying something, using facial expressions, or by some other action. The key to remember is that if there is no actual physical contact, then actions of others cannot possibly affect you, let alone hurt you. The Human Operators member is so self -aware that whatever other people do or say, they can react in the best possible way: by not changing overall mental status or emotions.

All information received from other people needs to be evaluated for importance or merit. Whatever the appreciate action is, it will have a higher chance of being the best decision if complete self-awareness is present. The most important aspect of this rule is that if there is no physical contact, then the way you feel should not be altered. If you are hit, then feel free to react; but if there is no contact, then there should not be any change in your mental state.

Minimize The Downtime

Of course, there are exceptions – when devastating news about the loss of life is heard, then any emotion or feeling is accepted. Remember the thought that "life is short" – feel as bad as you need, but not too long. Minimize the "downtime" that your brain needs to experience so you can create a happy and enjoyable life.

13-You are the gatekeeper of your own brain

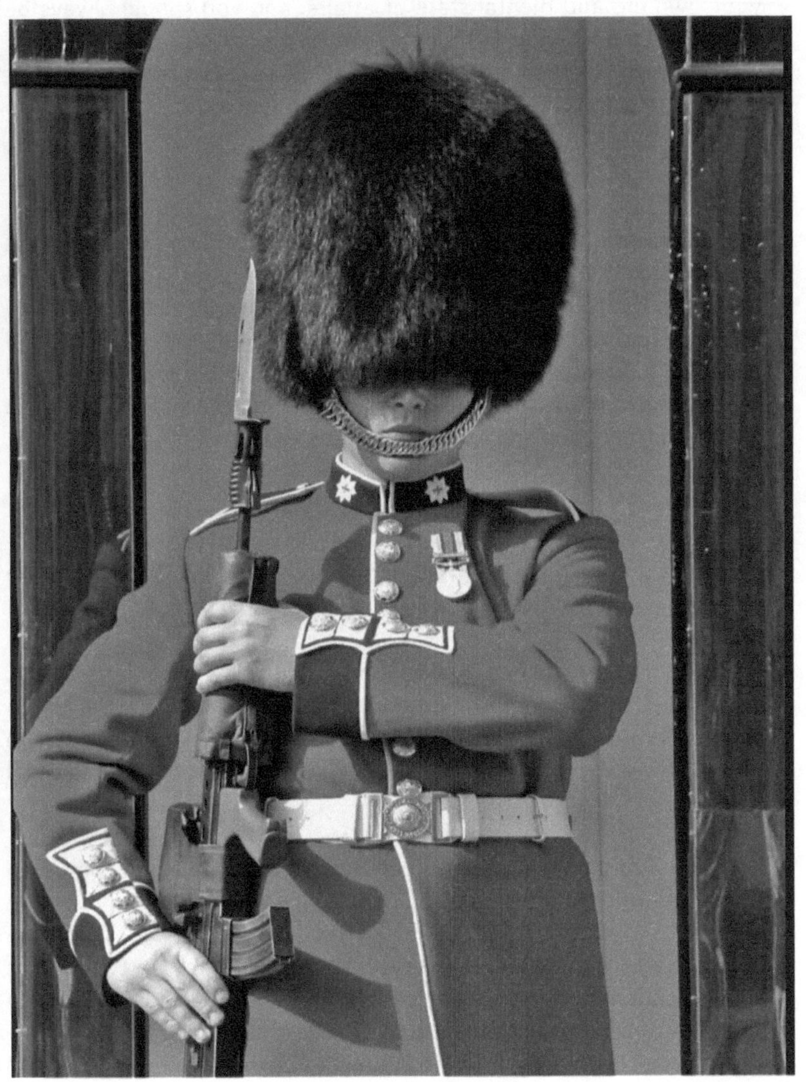

The gatekeeper has one job: only the good are allowed to pass through the gates. Nothing that will cause a problem is allowed through. Some gatekeepers are so good that only super-beneficial people or ideas are allowed into their life. You are the gatekeeper of your own life and mental state of affairs, and you should always be aware of who or what is trying to get past your gates. Evaluate all relationships for their positive, neutral, or negative effects on your mental state and create a Scoreboard of Influence.

Scoreboard of Influence

A Scoreboard of Influence can be made for your life by creating a list of all people that have an influence on you and observing them. Keep the list to the top twenty. The next step is to simply evaluate each of these people as to how they affect your mental state. Positive and negative influences should be easy to identify. Neutral people will require more thought and focus, as their influence may switch back and forth from good and bad, or just have very little impact.

Human Experiments

Below is a weeklong experiment exposing the influence of other people on your psyche.

Evaluate your mental health on a Sunday night. Try to be as specific as possible. Identify the positive people in your life. If possible, try to spend as much time with these people over the next week. Write down how each of these positive influences adds to your mental health.

At the end of the week, write down how your mental state compared to your mental state the week before. Take a week off.

Evaluate your mental health on a Sunday night. Try to be as specific as possible. Identify the negative people in your life. If possible, try to spend as much time with these people over the next week.
Write down how each of these influences detracts from your mental health. At the end of the week, write down how your mental state compared to your mental state the week before.

Analyze The Data

It is impossible to avoid all of the negative people in day to day life, so use the information that was just found to garner awareness of what positive influences offer, and what negative influences take away. Try to analyze specific reasons to how a positive person adds to your mental health. Concentrate on that in order to absorb it as much as possible. This is a time to be completely selfish. Absorb as many positive vibrations or feelings as possible, and truly relish in the emotional aftermath. On the flip side, also try to analyze specific reasons why a negative person detracts to your mental health. Concentrate on those elements to deflect the negative vibrations as much as possible.

Absorb the Good

The bottom line is: absorb as much good and deflect as much bad as you can. This will keep your mental world at neutral or better, and will probably edge towards improvement a great percent of the time.

14-Hearsay and third party information should be vetted personally before it is acted upon

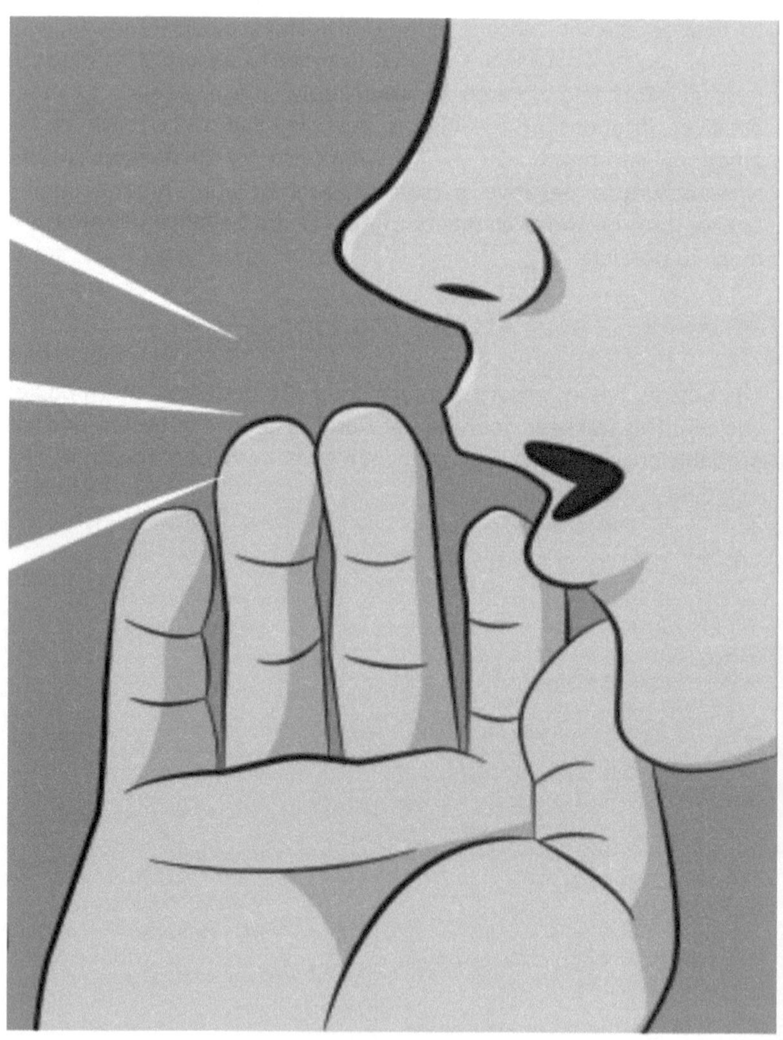

The mind and body can be calm and life can be enjoyable when information regarding important matters are known and verified. Uncertainty around other people and their motivations, statements, actions, and so on, can cause the mind to have all sorts of doubt and apprehensions. This type of mental activity should be avoided at all costs. Everyone likes to engage in potentially frivolous talk and gossip, and sometimes their discussion of "facts" are 100% wrong. All third party information should be considered suspect until verified personally.

Trust but Verify

During the Cold War between The Soviet Union and The United States there came a time when both counties had to start trusting the other in regards to the nuclear weapons each country was suppose to have. We trusted the other side, but the facts needed to be verified. So, each country sent inspectors to verify what was being said. This was a very successful system and should be copied in day to day life.

Haste Could Create Disasters

Take no action regarding third party information until you have verified the accuracy and source. No matter how upsetting the information is, never act until the information is found to be accurate. The consequences of acting before the information is vetted could be devastating to the mental wellbeing of the sometimes-fragile psyche. Look before you leap. Verify first. This may be as easy as one phone call, or as difficult as a spy novel, but always take the time to verify.

Stop Gossip Before It Starts

The absolute best case scenario is to just stop anyone from offering up gossip or third party information in the first place. If they must offer the information, immediately get on the phone and talk directly to the original source. You should ask something like this: "So and so says this about this, is this true?" To be Neutral or Better humans need to know that that life is short and information needs to be vetted as quickly as possible. No time should be wasted by being unsure about anything. Go to the source – immediately!

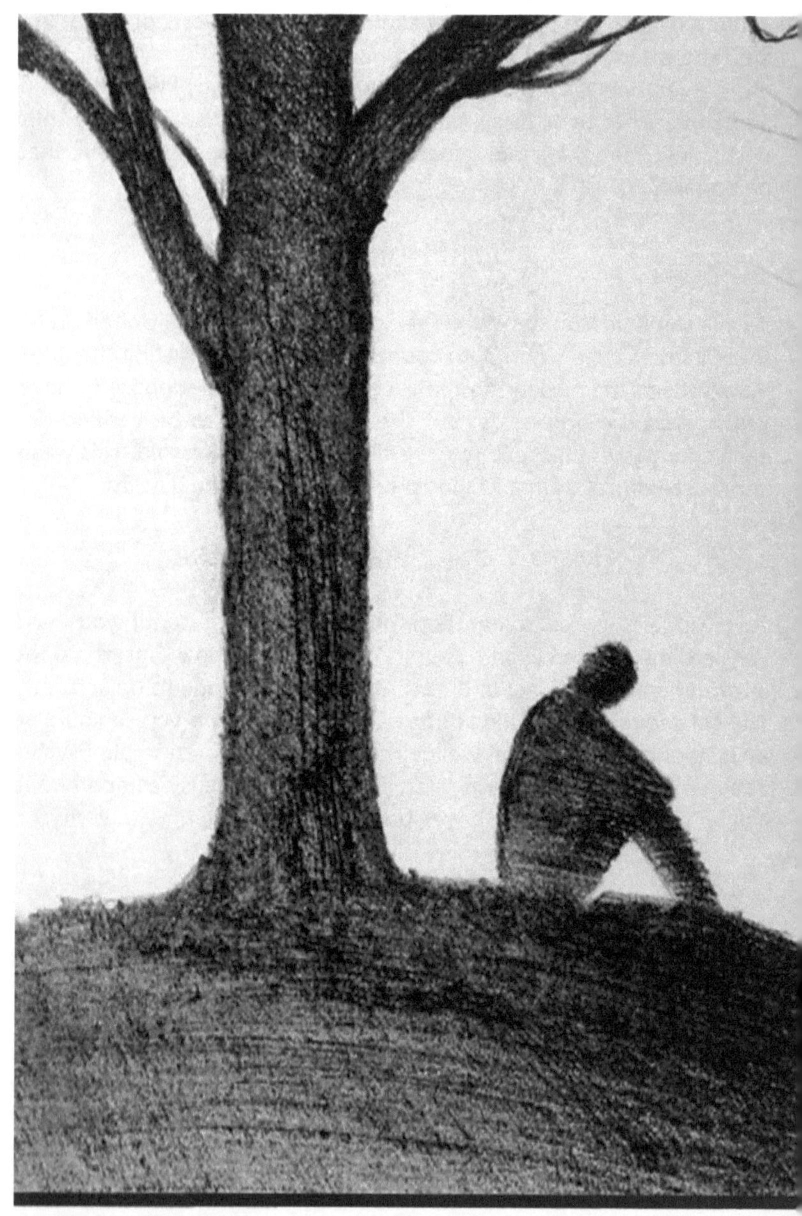

A human life can become a living hell when suddenly a loved one leaves or dies. How much of "a hell" is determined by the degree of dependency that existed on the human who is no longer available. If the dependency is deep, then prepare for weeks, maybe months if not years of pain. A deep throbbing pain in the chest and just an overall terrible feeling is the result of a deep grief over a loss. What can be done? What could shorten this grief period? Should the grief period even be shortened? If the grief period is shortened artificially could this cause permanent damage? A Neutral or Better state of mind knows that grief is important, but being neutral is always healthier then sinking into a deep dive of depression.

Maintain Control of Your Brain

Humans don't realize the control they have over their own brains. Grief is truly just feeling sorry for oneself as the reality of not having the human who has either died or physically vacated the area. Women live for grief, while men avoid it. Does mean men are heartless? No, it just equates that a high percentage men are programmed differently for reasons of survival. Just imagine this scenario: a darken cave lit by a single torch. A cavewoman howls with sadness over the death of their cave child. Does the caveman join her in this grief? He may want to, but he just can't. Why? Because at the entrance of the cave are three hungry wolves ready to eat both of them. The man cannot afford to wallow in grief, or everyone dies. It's pretty simple. Women are more prone to deep grief because their brains are programmed to "super bond" with any children they may produce. A human child can usually only survive if the mother devotes her entire soul to the child. This is why women have the capacity to go so deep and why their grief is deeper and last longer. All men have to do is kill the saber tooth tiger. No deep emotions here, just an ego that says, "I need to survive and I will figure out a way."

Being Aware of the Grief

So to help the grieving process in our modern society, the simple process of being self-aware at all times while being alive may indeed shorten the grief period from any major loss.

Lucky humans who have bonded with a spouse, sibling or any other human are allowed to grieve for the loss of this connection. The grieving can last a second or for a lifetime. The determining factor is how self-aware is the grieving party? A Neutral or Better state of mind is completely self-aware and can analyze grief on a daily basis. If the human is aware of the grief, then it can be managed. If the human is oblivious to the grief, then that human may wallow in this non-productive period for an eternity. Self-aware humans know grief is coming, so they are mentally prepared when grief arrives.

Avoid The Black Hole of Grief

Neutral or Better humans are so self-aware that they practice dealing with grief at low levels to prepare for the major events. The major events of life can throw a human consciousness into a deep black hole that some never return from. Self aware humans would rather enjoy life than to drop below neutral dragged there by grief.

If the human is unlucky enough to be responsible for the death of a loved one, then there is no way to shorten that grief. This type of grief is uncharted waters and may never be resolved. The only advice being Neutral or Better can offer in this situation is to make sure an argument never happens in a moving car, near a vehicle that is running, close to a second story or higher window, while there are guns in the area, that there is a solid fence around a pool, never passes large trucks at night on desert highways and any other possible situation where a stupid death can occur to anyone. A Neutral or Better brain sees all possibilities because being self-aware also involves a complete understanding of the surroundings.

Evolutionary Brain

Once a human achieves being Neutral or Better they know that a devastating loss is just a challenge. The software in the human brain sets up these grief scenarios and asks this question: is your type of brain "mush" or is this the type of brain that will be used in the "next evolutionary step of humanity." Maybe this question is mute since there are so many humans now, who cares if a percentage is not functioning to their highest potential due to grief.

Some grief or depressions may need drugs to manage, but a Neutral or Better mind is aware of its grief and depression, so they tend to try to manage their own brain chemistry.

The Bottom Line on Grief

Humans only have one life and if they chose to "grieve it" away, then go for it. **Neutral or Better** humans realize that they do truly only have one life, so they grieve for a reasonable amount of time and then get back to enjoying the only life available.

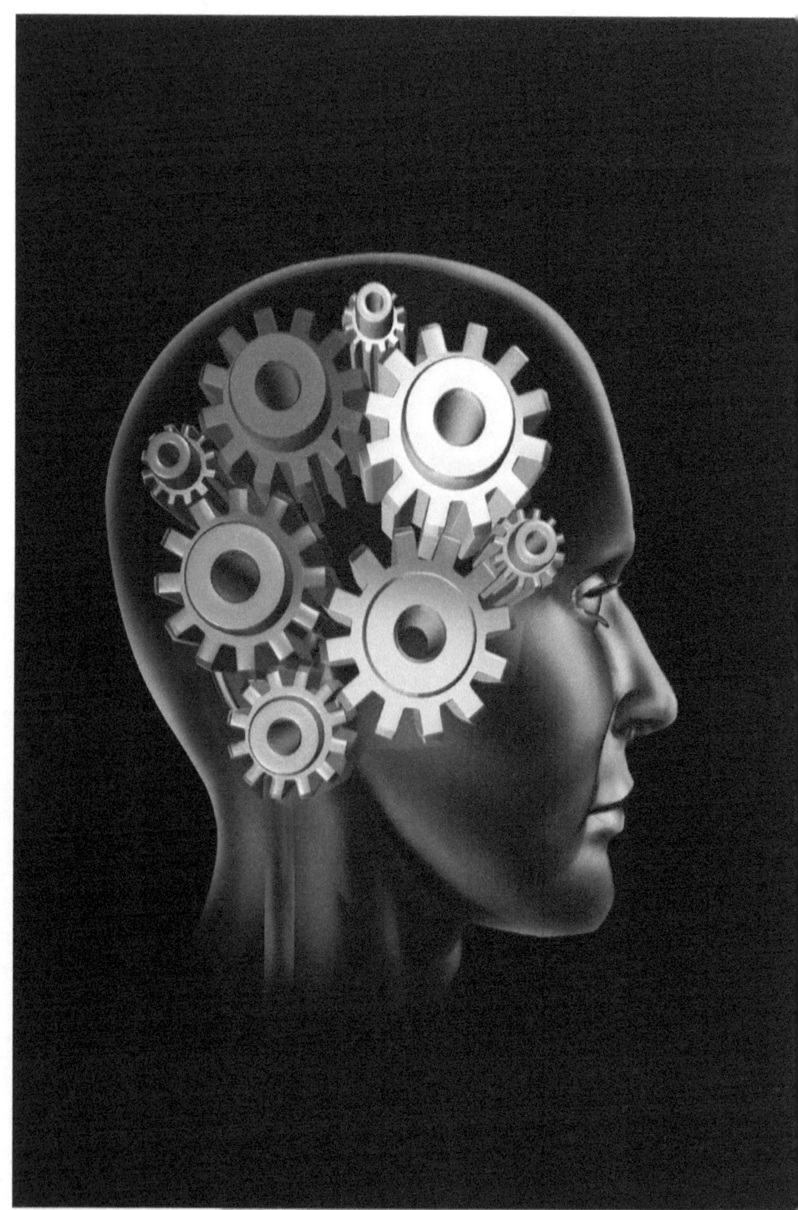

Indian Legend

There is an old Indian legend about God and how he handled a very important dilemma he was facing. To help solve this problem, God gathered up all the animals of creation for a meeting. As God stood before an animal of every shape and size, he thought deeply about this dilemma. He finally looked up the animals and started to explain," My friends, I'm in a deep quandary and I need your help. As you know my creation, he puts up finger quotes "man" is very clever animal, almost too clever. Anyway, I need to hide; he uses finger quotes again, "the secrets of life" from man until he's truly ready to receive them. If he finds them too soon, there could be a lot of additional trouble and I just can't handle that at the moment." All the animals agree as they know that man is nothing but trouble, all of the time. God continues," My dilemma is to determine the best hiding place for the secrets of life. I fear there is no place I can hide this from man." So, I need your help on this. Ideas? Anyone?

The Eagle Has the Answer

The animals talk among themselves until the strongest of the Eagles steps forward. "I have the answer!" the eagle yells out. "I will fly the secrets to the highest mountain top, because you know I'm the only one that can do that. Man will never find the secrets there. Man is worthless!" God seems to agree with the last statement and starts to think about the mountaintop, "That's a wonderful suggestion, but man is a clever thing, and he would eventually find the secrets there. Thank you very much Eagle." The eagle nods his head in agreement and moves backs into the group. More talking and then a giant whale is next to step up. "I have the answer!" says the giant whale. "I will take the secrets to the deepest part of the deepest ocean. Man will never think to look there or ever have the ability." God ponders the concept for a moment, but eventually shakes his head "no." God responds to the whale, "I like the way you think, but man is very clever and he will find the secrets in the deepest ocean. Thank you whale." The whale bows his head and moves back into the crowd. After a few moments, a huge badger steps forward. "I have the answer!" yells the badger. "I know where to hide the secrets; I will dig the deepest hole into the earth and bury the secrets there. No one will ever find them! No one!" God stamps a foot on the ground to check how stable the earth is and is almost convinced, but starts to shake his head again. "Excellent idea Mr. Badger, but unfortunately for all of us, man will find the secrets there; thank you." The badger steps back into the crowd.

God Is Pleased

Suddenly God's face lights up as if the answer is now clear. He turns and walks away from the crowd. The animals are confused and yell out to god. "Did you find the answer? Are you giving up?" God stops and turns back to the animals and apologizes and explains that the badger had given him an idea and he was so excited he was overwhelmed with happiness. God then walks closer to the group and says, "I have decided to hide the secrets of life in the one place man will never think to look. I will hide the secrets deep inside man himself; he will never ever think to look there." The animals all shake their heads in agreement and the group breaks up and they all go their separate ways. God is extremely happy.

The Spirt Dwells Within

Many religions and cultures discuss the concept that god is within every human and that "the spirit dwells" in every man and so on. What if this was just "code" that there is more inside every human then anyone could imagine? What if everything humanity would ever need to know for its entire existence was already imbedded in every human brain? When this concept is dwelled upon for a few minutes, there is nothing in life more powerful. Convincing a consciousness that everything that any human needs or wants to understand is already present in that brain is magical. The Human Operators member relishes in the concept that no matter what is needed as far as knowledge the information already exist in his or her brain. Now, the information needs to be accessed and that does require a little work. All the information in the universe is stored in every human brain and the key to this knowledge is determining how it is to access this information. Certain types of motivation are the key in accessing this data. A few motivations, such as "extinction," seem to be a super motivator. The knowledge discovered when real survival is on the line has been humanity's finest hour as far as searching for particular answers to particular impossible questions.

Two Evil Empires

When the United States was faced with extinction from two evil empires in World War II (Japan and Germany) a large number of brains started searching for the answer of salvation and those answers were the equations to atomic power. Two hundred and fifty thousand scientists and engineers were told that The American Way was at risk and we all may not survive unless they search their brains for the answers. After three years and a few billion dollars those scientists and engineers found the answers that saved The American Way from evil and destruction as they split the atom. Point a gun at a human's eyeball and the most amazing knowledge will just pop out.

Path to Space Travel

When the United States faced extinction from the evil empire of the Soviet Union, a lot of brains started searching for the answers of salvation and those were the equations to landing a man on the moon. Four hundred thousand scientists, engineers and technicians were told that The American Way was at risk and we all may not survive unless they search their brains for the answers. After seven years and a few billion dollars, those scientists and engineers found the answers that saved The American Way from evil and destruction and they landed a human on the moon. Point a gun at a human's eyeball and the most amazing knowledge will just pop out.

No Excuses!

This scenario has been played out millions of times throughout the course of humanity. So the bottom line on the human brain is that when the motivation is high enough, anything a human can imagine is possible. If a human brain or brains can split an atom and land on the moon, then day to day first world problems are a walk in the park. Neutral or Better humans know that when the motivation is strong enough than any knowledge can be discovered in their own brains.

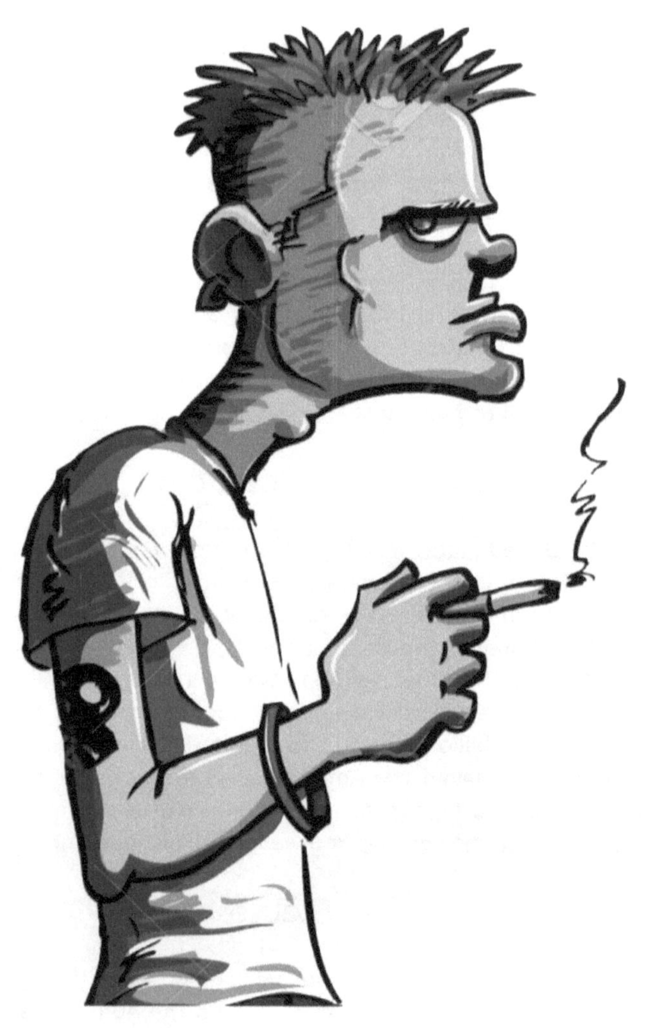

Neutral or Better means always being self-aware. Being self-aware also provided the ability to see drama before it even begins to develop. Most humans react in several different ways to drama directed at them, but when you are Neutral or Better you can use drama as entertainment.

Watch The Drama Flow

Yelling is the trademark of the un-aware and drama filled human. Whenever another human goes into drama mode – just take a step back and watch. DO NOT ENGAGE the drama filled human!! The drama filled human will go on autopilot and the drama will just flow out from them. Let them yell and scream and jump up and down, but DON'T ENGAGE. Just watch them and occasionally tweak your facial expression into a "are you crazy" expression. Eventually, the drama filled human will stop due to exhaustion. After a moment of silence, just ask one simple question, "Are you done?"

Imagine a Silent Film

The key to this type of exchange is that the Neutral or Better human never lets the drama filled human spark any emotions. No matter what anyone is accused of, the words of the drama filler human are not heard until the volume and the tone returns to normal. Just imagine a silent film with no audio at all, just the screaming actress or actor. The advanced self aware human even adds in the old time piano music to accompany the diatribe of the drama filled human. This is how to be entertained by a drama creator. When the show is over a rational discussion may take place or not.

18-Do not fear death
Fear a stupid death

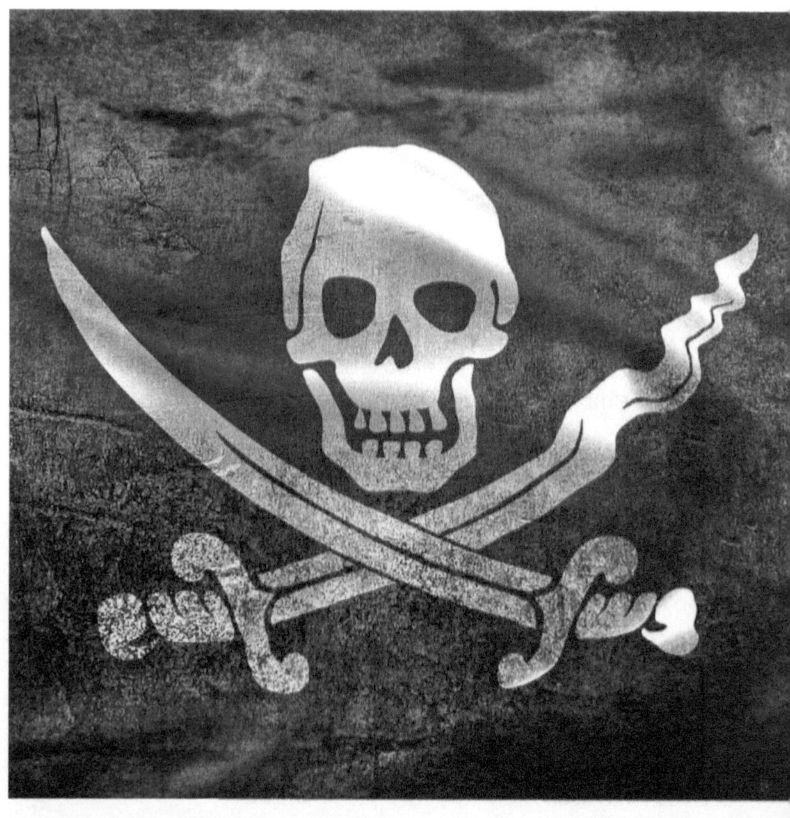

Death is part of life, but a stupid death is just stupid and only unaware humans end up dead due to simply being stupidity. Being Neutral or Better offers most humans the ability to be so self-aware that all situations are thoroughly vetted. When you are super self aware you see into the future and can spot a hazardous situation before it even begins. You are always checking the news and listening about other humans who were not self-aware and were so caught up in the moment that they didn't realize that they were about to die due to being stupid. The Darwin Awards track this "type" of human. Life is short; don't squander years of life by not being self-aware – all the time.

Only True Danger

The news media is constantly trying to scare viewers, because in reality that is their job. Being afraid of everything creates viewership. The list of potential dangers presented by the news media is very long. The list ranges from terrorism to gang murders, but there is truly only one danger we all face and that is from the cars we drive. We will not die from a terrorist bomb, we will not die from AIDS or Coronavirus, we will not die in an airliner crash or from a drug overdose. Humans in the year 2020 and beyond only face true danger when driving at 80 miles per hour in our tiny metal boxes.

So mitigate this risk there are several steps to take to insure your safety on the road; never drink and drive, never trust any other drivers to do the right thing and always assume other drivers don't see you at all. When changing lanes on the freeway don't assume that open space will stay open. Assume some other drivers also wants that same space and slowly move there. Whenever you are late for an off-ramp never make drastic and sudden moves to make that off-ramp. Always go to the next exist ramp. Making sudden moves of any types on the freeway is a recipe for disaster. Always drive safe, driving is truly the only danger we face and driving defensively will provide all the amazing years of life you were originally allocated.

Crossing The Street at Night

Accidents between cars driven by humans are very tough on the human body. Accidents between cars and an unprotected human body on the street are usually absolutely deadly for the human.

Autos traveling at 40 mph crush the human body. Flesh, bone and blood are rearranged in the most destructive way possible. At night driver's vision is 30% of vision during the day. This is a recipe for death and destruction. When walking at night be diligent that you are in danger of being killed by a passing auto. Do not trust drivers to see you at night. Yes, if you do get hit the accident will be their fault, but you'll be dead. So, who's the loser?

If you have to walk or run at night on the street, even if you are just crossing a highway to going to a bar or restraint, the danger exists. If you park down the block and across the street to avoid paying valet fees and then get hit and killed or your wife or child get hit or killed, is saving $10 worth it?

History of Failure

History is packed full of failures when the the worst case scenario was not addressed, especially when there might have been someone sounding the alarm. Engineers who made the solid rocket boosters for the Space Shuttle were sounding the alarm when the temperature went far below accepted levels. No one listened and the shuttle literarily blew up in 1986. Years of warnings about pandemics went on deaf ears before January 2020, but the entire human population was put in harms way and thousands died worldwide. Warnings regarding German aggression in 1930 were ignored and seventy-two million humans had died when World War Two finally ended. Middle East experts warned that without a plan invading Iraq would cause tremendous chaos afterwards. The warnings were correct as the terrorist group ISIS emerged after the Americans left and thousand more died.

Always take time to listen to warnings from anyone around you and especially from your gut instinct. If there is a possible danger, a second look with not hurt and just may save years of suffering.

When you are in a **Neutral or Better state of mind,** you always see the worse case scenario in every situation. Don't lose years of your life or loved ones just because all the possible scenarios were not evaluated. Take nothing for granted and expect the unexpected.

19-Abandon drama relationships

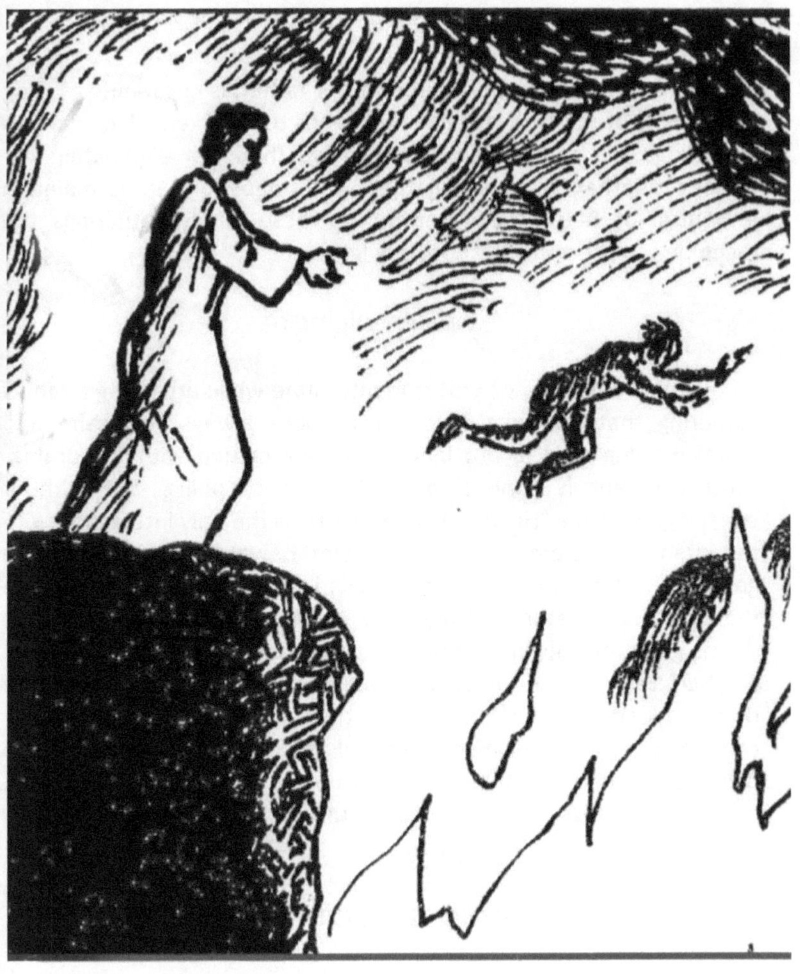

Life is short and becoming Neutral or Better humans need to reflect on this fact every day. Life is so short that dealing with other humans that constantly inflicting mental strain could shorten an already short life. To become Neutral or Better humans need to evaluate the humans in their lives and slowly eliminate the drama producing ones from their existence. Even close family members can be eliminated according to the rules of being Neutral or Better.

Eliminate People - Even Parents

 If a family member, even the mother or father, is constantly causing drama 50% of the time, then action needs to be taken. Since parents or siblings are part of family gatherings then just eliminating the father or mother from these gatherings is impossible. So, to maintain a Neutral or Better mind set during these family gatherings the technique to use is called "Cordially Ignore."

Cordially Ignore

To maintain a Neutral or Better mental state while attending a family gathering that normally erupts into chaos always stay calm and practice being cordial, but ignore. The interaction with the drama-causing parent is conducted by being very polite, but without engaging. A simple "Hello – How are you?" is the only interaction with the drama generator. From that point onward during the entire gathering – there is no interaction. Avoid sharing the same space with the drama generator – always smile but never engage. When the drama generator begins to cause trouble just stand back and observe. NO NOT ENGAGE!! An important point to make is to not blame the drama generator for the problems they cause because they really can't help themselves. Being Neutral or Better is to know not to blame any human for their actions. Humans do the best they can. A calm mind realizes when another human's best is trouble for for everyone else.

Stress from Religions, Societies and Cultures

Religions, societies and cultures stress that parents are important to take care of, but if one or more parent are the cause of your unhappy life, then cut the cord. Rules and regulations from these three institutions are very helpful in the keeping order in the societies we exist in, but they should not be the source of our demise. If the relationships to parents, siblings or other relatives need to be severed then cut them as soon as possible.

Cutting The Cord

Anyone can either cut the cord to relatives completely by eliminating these destructive humans physically or mentally. Once the cord is cut the prevailing attitude will be, "Why did I wait so long to this?"

Physically removing yourself from the vicinity of the destructive parents is the easiest way to cut the cord. There can be many very good and true excuses to move far away or at least a two-hour distance; new job, new husband or wife, doctor's orders, school and so on. A two-hour drive will drastically reduce the time spent with the destructive parent or parents and allow for a much easier mental life.

From God to Just a Human

A Neutral or Better state of mind realizes that the operator of a human body should always make choices for their best interest at heart and loyalties to other humans that are detrimental need to altered.

To mentally cut the cord will require some practice, but will serve you in other areas of your life if successful. By design, parents dominate a child's life, but when the child's self-awareness develops enough for the child to realize that the parent is no longer an asset, then mental actions need to be taken. The respect and reverence for a parent is still embedded deep in the brain, but the actions and words of the parent can now be discounted. Words and actions of parents are so important to children because the parent is the "god" to the child. This worshipper -god relationship lasts as long as it does, but the imprint has been made, and if the parents are always supportive and helpful, then the worshipper-god relationship can continue forever. In the case where the god or the parents are now causing pain and suffering, then the child needs to alter their opinion of the parent from god to just another human. Once the parent has been relegated to just another human status, then their actions and words can be dealt with as any other distraction. You can continue your love for a parent, but the destructive ties will be severed and the mental state of the child will be free to enjoy life and deal with unexpected drama more easily.

 Once a child has eliminated the "god status" of a parents, then this technique can be used for any other human who might be inflicting drama in your life. Simply put, to elevate yourself mentally to equality with any other human will offer a stronger platform to live your life. To elevate your mental status with any other human who at one time you thought was superior is a groundbreaking moment. Life among other humans is a constant negotiation.   When you can participate in any negotiations from a position of equality, then the results of your give and take will be much more satisfying. Elevating a negotiation to human to human instead of child to god will supply years of a calm mind and a gateway to answers to questions not yet asked.

20-Never lash out at anyone!

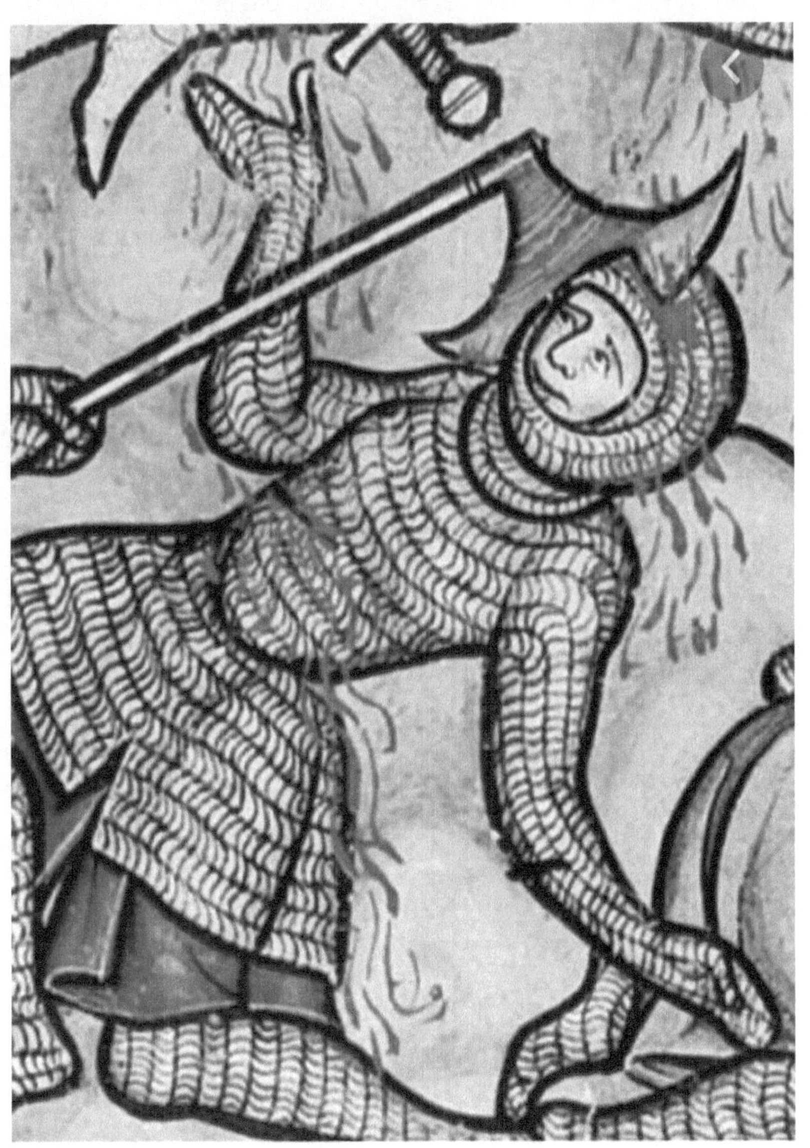

When life dishes up anything that might cause outrage never lashing out and anyone will keep the Neutral of Better state of mind. The cliché is to count ten seconds and the react, but in this new world the counting continues until much later.

Vent in a Vacuum

Self aware humans use an opportunity like this to vent and the venting needs to be done in a vacuum where no other human ever sees or hears it. Being Neutral or Better offers a few options in this regard.

Expressing Outrage

The first is to write a letter to the other human to express the outrage. This letter is never in emailed, this letter is always handwritten. The letter is the foulest and vile letter ever written between two human beings. The offended human calls out the other human and reduces their existence to less than the slime in the gutter. This letter is so off the wall that small children would start crying if it was read to them. The language used is disgusting and littered with F-bombs and as many cuss words s possible.

Insanity

This letter may even sound as if written by an insane human with the express intent of bodily harm to anyone in the vicinity. When the letter is finished the letter is reread several times. If the offended is alone, he or she may even read the letter out loud a few times. The purpose of this entire action is to drain any feeling of being insulted out of your system.

Burning The Outrage

After the letter is read enough times the offended human will tear up this letter into several small pieces and then the pieces will be burned. As the smoke raises and dissipates so does any outrage that be left.

If any outrage still lingers, then a second letter even worse than the first needs to be written and the same schedule is followed. Once all the outrage has flowed out the widow with the smoke then a civilized response can be offered or none at all. member knows that the only way to get out of a hole is to stop digging.

Always Handwritten

The fore mentioned letter is always handwritten because there can never be a chance that a letter of this type is sent by mistake.

21-Neutral or Better Time Machine

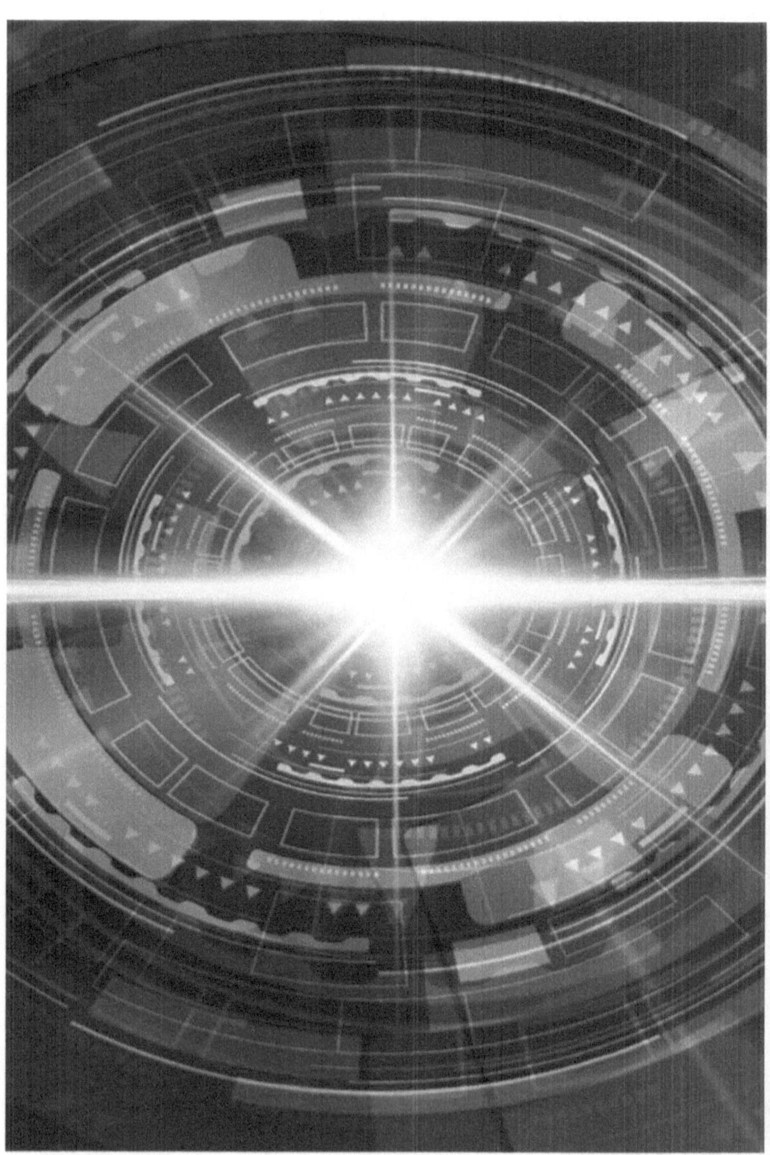

How is it possible to maintain a **Neutral or Better** frame of mind when a terrible, awful unpleasant task awaits you? Examples could be a long tortuous drive, a weekend stay with the in-laws, writing a book or making five hundred phone calls to sell something when it's possible 498 of those phone calls will yield a "never call my again" response. Yes, a journey of a thousand miles begins with the first step, but what if you could finish before you even started?

Propelled into The Future

The Neutral or Better Time Machine is available whenever its needed and the machinery is as simple as imagination. As soon as the task at hand is deemed a chore or an event that will be a horrible experience, then just turn on the time machine. The Neutral or Better Time Machine instantly catapults any human to the exact moment in the future when the task is totally completed. Maybe even hours after when a celebration is taking place or on the drive home or any moment that will be enjoyable. Firmly plant your conscious mind at the glorious moment for just a few seconds. Imagine how that moment will feel. Imagine what relief that instant in time will generate. After enjoying that future moment, get back to work and then let real time just catch up to you in that magical moment in the future.

Share The Time Machine

When this technique is mastered, the annoying task and the time that is required to accomplish the task go by in the blink of an eye. This is a distractionary mind game and nothing else. This technique is best used with a fellow worker. Explain about the time machine and how this magical moment in the future when the work is done is occupying your thoughts. They will think you are crazy, but when that moment in the future does come and you announce that "see – here we are!" your fellow worker will see how fun the Time Machine is.

22- Love and being Neutral or Better

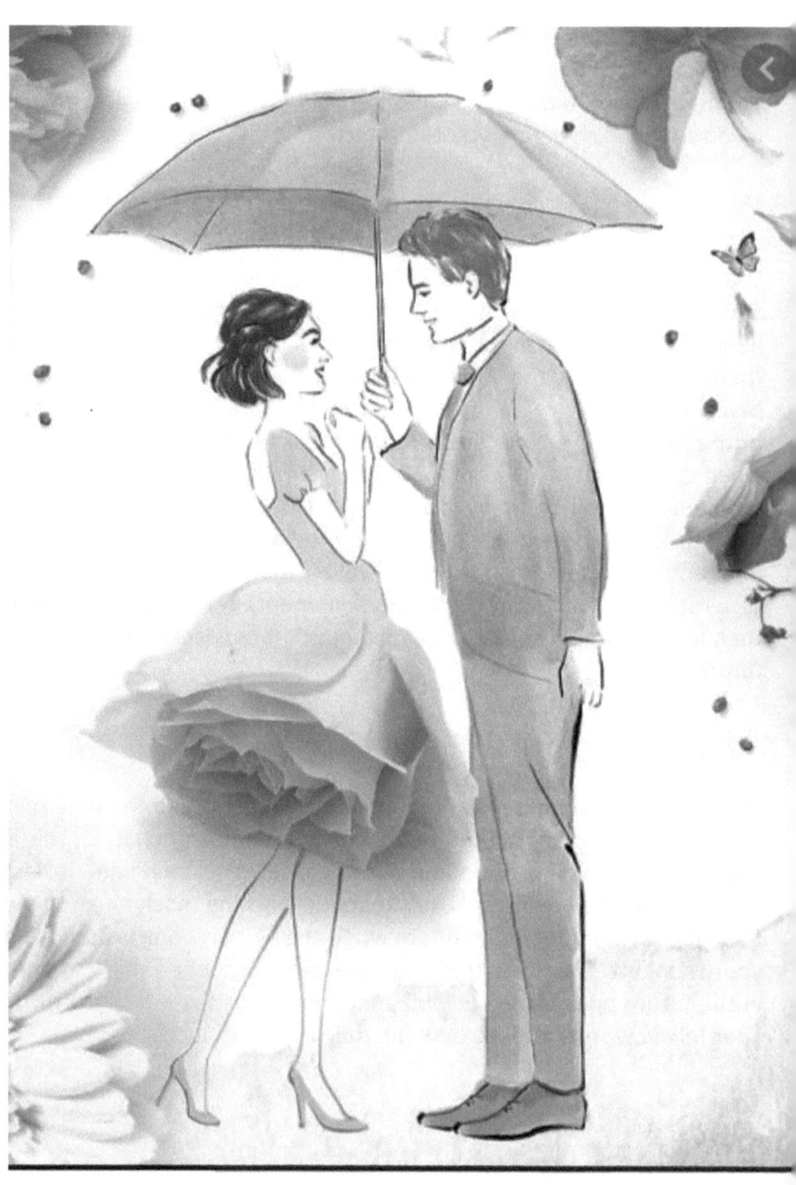

Love has been acted upon, talked and written about ever since caveman #1 whacked caveman #2 over the head because they were both after cavewoman #3. LOVE: why does a human want or need it? Why does it cause so much trouble? What is the real purpose of love?

Love Equals Survival

 The simple answer is that love equals survival. The more love in one's life the better the survival chances. The more people that love you your chances living a longer life increase. If an infant's mother did not love that child, then that child is in deep trouble. In a Neutral or Better state of mind the human knows that love is a powerful force and that awareness of the love emotion is deeply important.

Hardwired Love

A mother's love should be unconditional. Love for a child is hardwired in the female's brain and this is across all species. Try messing with a bear cub and watch the mother bear go berserk. This type of programming is paramount to the continuation of life in most warm-blooded mammals. Any species where the mother did not "love" the offspring then that species probably no longer exists.

A Neutral or Better human is aware that love equals survival. The more love you can generate from other humans the better chance of this survival. Self aware humans knows that no one owes you anything, so if love is offered and is not returned then there is no animosity, no hurt feelings or any other negative emotions. With hundreds, thousands and maybe even tens of thousands of fellow humans in the same general vicinity any type of love is available; it is just a matter of time and effort to find it and cultivate it.

Romantic Love

Romantic love can be an amazing asset to a Neutral or better state of mind. Romantic love begins with being completely self-aware of the three steps to love. The three steps are: 1) Attraction – 2) Trust – 3) The Conscious Decision to Become Dependent on that fellow human.

Yes, even though the outside world will fight tooth and nail regarding this fact, the self aware human knows that love equals dependency.

Three Steps to Love

The human brain has been programmed for love and love involves three distinct steps. Most humans have no clue about these steps because most humans run strictly on autopilot.

Step One - Step one is attraction and this can be in felt in an instant or can develop over time. What is attraction? Humans are attracted to other humans for many reasons which include; body shape, face, hair, voice, personality, status and so on. Attraction is an involuntary response just like breathing. Attraction just happens.

Step two – Step two Is trust and trust requires time to truly evaluate. Is your new partner truthful? Is your new partner consistence in what they say? Truth is very important due to your mental state in step number three.

Step three – Step three is when your brain decides to go completely dependent on this new human. You won't even know this is happening. One day you will wake up and be completely dependent. The dependency varies in intensity and can grow over time or completely disappear. When a relationship ends you'll know exactly how deep the dependency was by the time it requires to recover from the loss.

The Sex Storm

The human brain offers love for two main reasons. These reasons included survival and the hope that a sex storm will occur. As stated before the more love in a human's life, the better chances of survival. The human brain has created The Sex Storm between humans for one outcome and one outcome only and that outcome are as many new humans as possible.

Wildfire

Think of a sex storm like a wildfire storm. A human can feel it coming on with great anticipation. All three step of love are not needed for the sex storm to take place. As a matter of fact, none of the three steps of love are needed for a sex storm to happen. A sex storm is an 10overwhelm desire to have sex with another human and this storm can last five minutes or a lifetime. After the sex storm is over there could be as new human left to grow in the woman.

Eight Billion Living Humans

The number of living humans on planet Earth has been growing for approximately 10,000 years from five million to the present day eight billion. Pandemics and natural disasters may decrease the population but the one constant factor are the sex storms that humans go through. Without sex storms eight billion humans would just not be born. Sex storms even may start a relationship that lasts a lifetime.

```
aceAll(" ", " ", a);
a.split(" "); } $("#
array_from_string($
1(), c = use_unique(a
0))); if (c < 2 * b -
, this.trigger("clic
!= a[b] && " " !=
logged").val(); c = a
ength;b++) { -1 !=
; for (b = 0;b < c.l
("#User_logged").
ck(function().val(
```

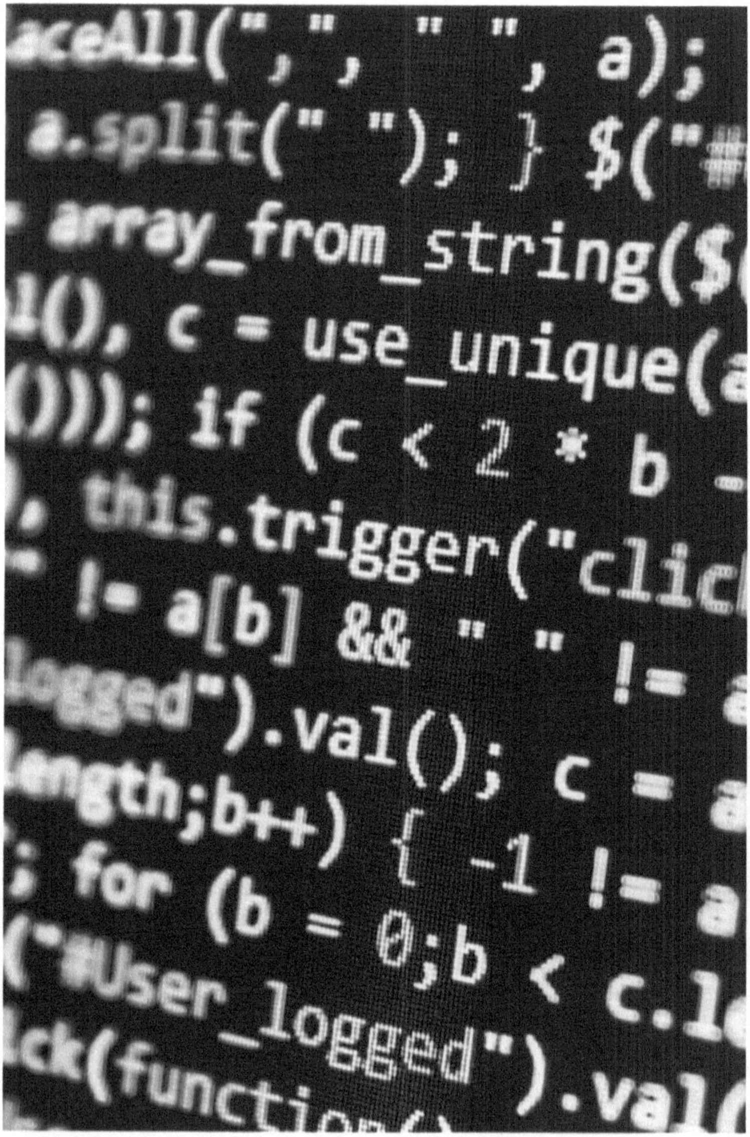

A woman who was molested five years ago still can't stop thinking about her experience. A soldier witnesses the horrors of war and relives those images every day. A child is involved in a car crash sees the destruction over and over. These conditions can be diagnosed as Post Traumatic Stress Disorder. These events on an esoteric level have corrupted lines of software code in the human brain.

Human Operating System

The human brain works just like a computer. As a matter of fact, the design of today's computer is an exact duplicate of the human brain. All computers have a basic operating system, which enables the computer to function and accept commands. The human brain is frontloaded with the software that manages the body from start to finish. This software in the human brain is completely responsible for keeping any human live, while the human operator truly only needs to fuel, rest and keep the body warm.

Corrupted Software

When the software code of any computer is corrupted, then those lines of code could disrupt all or part of the computer operation. PDSD type events can disrupt the operation of the brain, but only the self-aware portion. With PTSD the body still functions, cells are still dividing, muscles can still move bones, oxygen is still being processed through the lungs and about a million other operations are still happening. To realize this concept by the human with PTSD maybe the first step in overwriting bad code. If the human can realize that the brain is still working at a high level of efficiency, then the difficulties the human is having maybe diminished ever so slightly.

Brain Is Still Working

 The thought process may go something like this, "I know I'm screwed up since the accident, but my body is still working. There are a million commands my brain is sending and receiving every minute. My brain is still working. My life, my ability to function at all since birth has to be pure magic. Life is MAGIC, so I'm going to fix my own brain with magic."

This mantra may not fix anything, but being self-aware of the problem and having the PTSD sufferer acknowledge that his or her brain is still working magnificently may just start the process to recovery. A one percent improvement is an improvement.

Computer Repair

Disruptive lines of code need to be overwritten by other lines of code. Of course, this is easier said than done, but concentrating on replacing any code or thought in your head is an epic start. From this moment forward, whenever you are experiencing a negative thought, worry or anything that is not pleasant, immediately start to overwrite those thoughts with new ones. Overwrite the corruptive code with productive code. When destructive thoughts, "I do not have enough money," occur immediately replace them or overwrite this line of code with "how do I make more money?" This needs to happen immediately. The longer the negative thought exists, the more damage it can do. Being self-aware of what thoughts are doing to your state of mind is the key to this technique.

Overwrite the Bad Code

When you first sense a negative thought about anything, immediately overwrite that thought with the anti-virus thought. The sooner that code is overwritten the sooner you'll be ready to enjoy life because being alive is the baseline for happiness.

Institutions also provide code to overwrite negative thoughts. Society offers drugs and counseling to deal with PTSD. The drugs and counseling as far as the numbers are concerned are the most effective way to relieve a human from the pain and stress of PTSD. The medical community works exclusively on a percentage basis. If treatment is seen as successful on 51% of the population, then that is the treatment that is recommended. If a patient happens to be on the wrong side of that equation, then that patient needs to seek additional treatments.

Religions also offer new code to overwrite dysfunctional or defective programming. Drug and alcohol addicts write over these destructive codes with the code of a higher power with the famous 12-step program. Christianity and Buddhism are often used to sway an addict onto a new path. A PTSD patience may also find relief from the corruptive code by overwriting those impressions with these religious dogma, rules and regulations.

Jesus or The Universe Involved

Examining how these institutions offer help in this area it seems that having either Jesus or The Universe LOVE YOU may help to overwrite the defective code. Any human who feels completely lost may respond to the fact that these higher powers do care for them. After these higher powers are informed about a human's existence and their troubles that may just be the ticket for some relief. The bottom line is that who doesn't want at least one person to know and care about their problems. Who doesn't want a GOD or an entire universe to care about them?

The Canyon Exercise

PTSD is a major brain dysfunction and will probably not be solved by reading this book, but smaller less invasive brain problems might just be. The Canyon Exercise will offer some relief to smaller brain problems. This exercise is best practiced at night while in bed because it should calm your mind and put you to sleep. The Canyon Exercise begins with imagining the dysfunctional code causing a gap between happiness and peace. With this gap in place, there just is no peace. With this gap in place the mind cannot bridge the gap to a calm mind. So, the trick is to manually build a ladder to overcome this gap with love, either the love that Jesus has for you or the love that The Universe has for you or the love that you have for someone else or the love you have for yourself.

Mental Gap

Imagine a canyon. The size of the canyon will be determined by the size of the dysfunctional code. How big is the mental gap? How big is the problem? This exercise requires the exact problem to be determined and examined. Once you have determined the exact cause of the mental problem, then you can visualize the size of the canyon you have to climb out of. The problem will eventually be eliminated as the love from Jesus or the universe or the love you have for yourself, or someone else is used to build a ladder to the top. This could be a very slow process that might require months, if not years.

Love DNA

Building the ladder to the top of the canyon is not imaging building the ladder out of wood or steel, this ladder needs to be constructed out of *LOVE DNA*. To create this first step *LOVE DNA* needs to be understood. Once that term is defined, then the remaining steps can be created. *LOVE DNA* will not be easy to define – the meaning will be different for each individual. Examining your thoughts and emotions trying to determine what LOVE DNA means is time not spent lost in the destructive mental problem. PTSD is a preoccupation with an event or events that cause a very uneasy life, so anything that can take the place of this preoccupation is a positive thing.

Love Memory

Once LOVE DNA has been defined, then the rest of the steps of the ladder can be constructed. These steps can be created out of LOVE MEMORIES. To create each new step on the path to the top of the canyon will require a LOVE MEMORY to be recalled and analyzed. To analyze a LOVE MEMORY, all the details of that moment of LOVE need to be thoroughly embraced. The who, what, where, why and how of that LOVE MEMORY needs to be comprehended at the deepest level possible. Once that LOVE MEMORY has been understood, then the next step can be constructed with another LOVE MEMORY and so on and so on until the top of the canyon is breached.

Endless Steps – One at a Time

At the beginning of this journey to the top of the canyon there may have seemed an endless amount of steps required. As more and more LOVE MEMORIES are constructed the canyon may indeed become smaller and smaller.

The human brain is the most amazing machine in the universe. Taking control of its power could truly only be steps away.

24- Third Party Neutral Observer

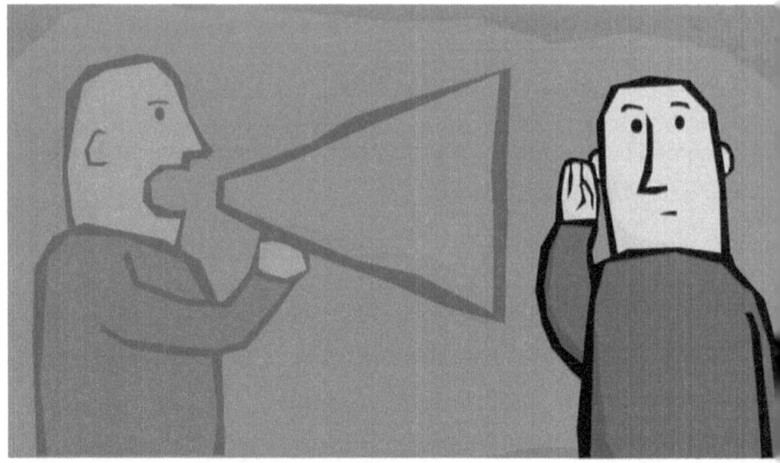

When you are faced with a decision and you just don't know what is the best way to go, it's time to bring out your Third Party Neutral Observer for some help.

Three Types of Neutral Observers

There are three types of Neutral Observers that are available; yourself, a respected human that you know and a respected human that you know about. The concept is to imagine this completely neutral third party sitting in the same room as you during negotiations.

Negotiations of any type are always full of emotions. Most conversations between humans involve some sort of negotiations concerning the next step. Some are completely meaningless as far as outcome, but a few do concern life and death situations.

Easy Exercise

Let's start with the easiest, non-consequential decisions and one third party neutral observer exercise that you perform already; the decision and negotiation on what to have for dinner.

Past Dinner Decisions and You

Imagine standing in the living room with another human, and the question of what to have for dinner becomes the topic of the conversation. To start this exercise, instantly start populating the room with your past self having dinner in four possible locations.   In the northeast corner of the room, imagine yourself eating dinner in your own kitchen. The "kitchen you" explains silently or out loud the virtues of staying at home. Now leave the "kitchen you" and inspect the "pizza parlor you" in another corner. You see the "pizza parlor you" and hear yourself describing what is best about this place. The food, the service whatever you remember as many details as possible is being conveyed by the "pizza parlor you." Now select two other eaters and place them in the remaining two corners. You have all the information with you to make an informed decision. The trick here is to hear yourself speak to you and help with the decisions. You may even ask yourself questions because this version of you is completely neutral. This "third party you" has no agenda and only delivers the true facts of all aspects of the last visit.

The Third Party You

Learn to extract as much information of the "third party you" as possible because he or she has all the details and facts that you have forget. Don't forget to ask about the aftermath of the dinner. How did the food settle an hour after dinner? How did your wallet like the dinner?

Learn to trust the "third party you" because he or she is void of emotions. The third party is strictly about the facts and a reasonable assessment regarding the outcome. The "Gut Feeling" may override the third party you, but at least you'll know that a stable true second onion is available.

Major Life Decisions

As the decisions become more intense and the outcome has more consequence, then the seriousness of the third party conversation becomes more important.

Let's chose an important decision such as cheating your spouse. Of course, if you cheat on your spouse all the time, then this conversation is mute. This type of third party conversation only works if this will be your first time cheating. Please place these four people in your third party conversation; your spouse, one close friend, yourself and the person you might soon be cheating with. It is much better to have this conversation when all parties are calm and non-emotional.

Third Party You – No Agenda

The best place to start is with your third party self. Have your third party self explain all the details of this action, the good and the bad. Then repeat these questions to everyone in the room. This is a good exercise even if you don't have a cheating partner in mind because if you are thinking about cheating, the situation will present itself and you'll be ready to make the best decision.

If you've cheated on your spouse before, then the conversation can include real experience from all parties.

Talking to the Dead - Third Party Conversations

Respect of a long-gone relative can go a long way in helping you make a decision. If you respected a close relative and enjoyed their advice while they were alive, then the advice can continue long after they have died. Place the relative in the room with you. Imagine this relative being the age where he or she gave you the best advice.

Have them start the conversation because they already know your situation? They will get right to the point and will waste no time.

To check their advice, bring in someone you had no respect for while they were alive and listen to them. Their advice should be the complete opposite.

Famous Third Party Advice

If you happen to be into history and have watched documentaries on famous people or have read biographies of humans of great stature living or not, then these humans can also help you with making the correct decisions.

After reading an in-depth reflection of Benjamin Franklins or Thomas Jefferson's life and philosophies, these great men's minds are now available to help with any decision making that might arise. Even though Mr. Franklin and Mr. Jefferson were not personal acquaintances, their thoughts and deeds are available to help guide a human with any problem they may face.

Research Life and Deeds

Before even starting to research on a famous person's life and deeds, if the concepts of helping with decision making in the future is the goal, then those moments will stand out during the research.

Famous people can also be used to agree with a decision already made. If your sure4 cheating on your spouse is a good thing, the bringing in President Kennedy to talk about his infidelities might push you over the cliff so to speak.

Learn from History's Mistakes

Famous humans have made all the decisions good and bad. Use their experiences to make a present-day life the best possible.

25- Lists of Truth

This is custom made for marriage problems, couples about to be married or any relationship

LOVE LIST

THINGS I LOVE ABOUT MY SPOUSE OR FUTURE SPOUSE

1)___________________________

2)___________________________

3)___________________________

4)___________________________

5)___________________________

6)___________________________

7)___________________________

8)___________________________

9)___________________________

10)__________________________

HATE LIST

THINGS I HATE ABOUT MY SPOUSE OR FUTURE SPOUSE

1)___________________________

2)___________________________

3)___________________________

4)___________________________

5)___________________________

6)___________________________

7)___________________________

8)___________________________

9)___________________________

10)__________________________

Humans join in all sorts of relationships and these relationships can be a wonderful experience or just pure hell.

Here is a simple way to evaluate a relationship and instantly know if this union should continue or be terminated without another moment wasted. Why waste time and money with a marriage counselor if the sessions won't change the underlying major problems. Why stay at a job when the future will not offer what is truly needed to fulfill your life's dreams? Why get married in the first place if deep rooted problems will surface eventually?

Four Lists Technique

If there is trouble in paradise and the marriage is on the rocks, use the Four List Technique to super evaluate how the relationship stands.

Separation and divorce have been mentioned and friends and family have suggested that marriage counseling has to be considered before anything drastic is done. Before making that first appointment with the counselor sit down with your spouse with four sheets of paper and two pens.

Two Lists Each

Each party will construct two lists. One list is ten things that you just love about your partner and then create a list of the ten things you hate about your partner.

When these list are complete, each party will read out loud the love list. This is a very important first step. If any of love lists contain zero items, then call the lawyers and start dividing up the assets. If there are ten items of love on both sides, that's a great start to this exercise and it is time to move on to the next step.

Absolutely Hate List

The second list are ten things that you absolutely hate about your partner. Try to make this list as detailed and exact as possible. There can be no gray areas. When complete, read these lists out loud.

Items on these lists may be well know or a complete surprise; this fact does not matter; what does matter is what happens next.

This is the time that the great negotiation begins and this negotiation will determine the life or death of the relationship.

The items on the "I Hate List" are discussed one at a time. One spouse can complete all of his or her items and then the next spouse can read his or her items. Or items can alternate between spouses. The wife reads item one and the husband reads his item one and so on.

Negotiation

Spouse number one reads the first **Hate List** item. Each item needs to be addressed by the spouse that is responsible for the hate items. For example, if the one if the items describe a lack of sex in the relationship then that item needs to be negotiated out to a mutual conclusion. There does need to be some give and take here, but if there can be no consensus on a negotiated agreement on this item, then walk away from this relationship immediately. Don't wait until weeks or months of counseling and money go to waste. Life is way too short.

No Sex

For example, if there is no sex in this relationship then this has to be negotiated out to a mutual agreement. Going from no sex to sex once per week or once per day needs to be addressed. Both parties need to find some middle ground. If the no sex spouse refuses to ever have sex, then the option of going outside the marriage is put on the table. If this is agreed upon then the details need to be worked out and put in writing. If any type of sex is opposed to by one if the spouse, then call the lawyers, this relationship is over.

Hate List

Other items could be one spouse hates the other spouse's friends or one spouse is too messy, or a spouse may be too fat or is angry or bitchy or unpleasant to be around or never shows any type of affection or religious affiliation. These all have to be negotiated out to a mutual conclusion. If one of the items on the I Hate List is that that spouse truly hates the other spouse, then call the lawyers.

There could also be problems with the way children are raised. Now, this is an item where the child's future is the most important.   This is where research is needed by both parents. Adults in your day to day life that both spouses respect in as many ways as possible need to be talked to. These adults are then interrogated in regards to how there were raised. There are many items to explore, but again this is a matter of negotiation and if there is no progress on negotiation, then call the lawyers.

Removing an Item

Negotiations can take the form of agreeing to one item and removing another item completely from the list. If an item from the hate list is removed, then it can never be bought up again to your spouse or internally. It has to be let go completely.

Contract for Later Reference

All items on each the hate list need to be addressed and negotiated. When all items on both lists have been negotiated out and both parties are happy with the results, then all negotiations need to be written down in a contract. This contract needs to be signed by both parties and now this contract is the go to for any further problems. All the agreed upon solutions have to be in the contract. If there are future disputes, then the contract needs to posted in a well traveled spot in the home for easy reference.

CONCLUSIONS

Time to turn off the AUTOPILOT

For Individuals and Humanity

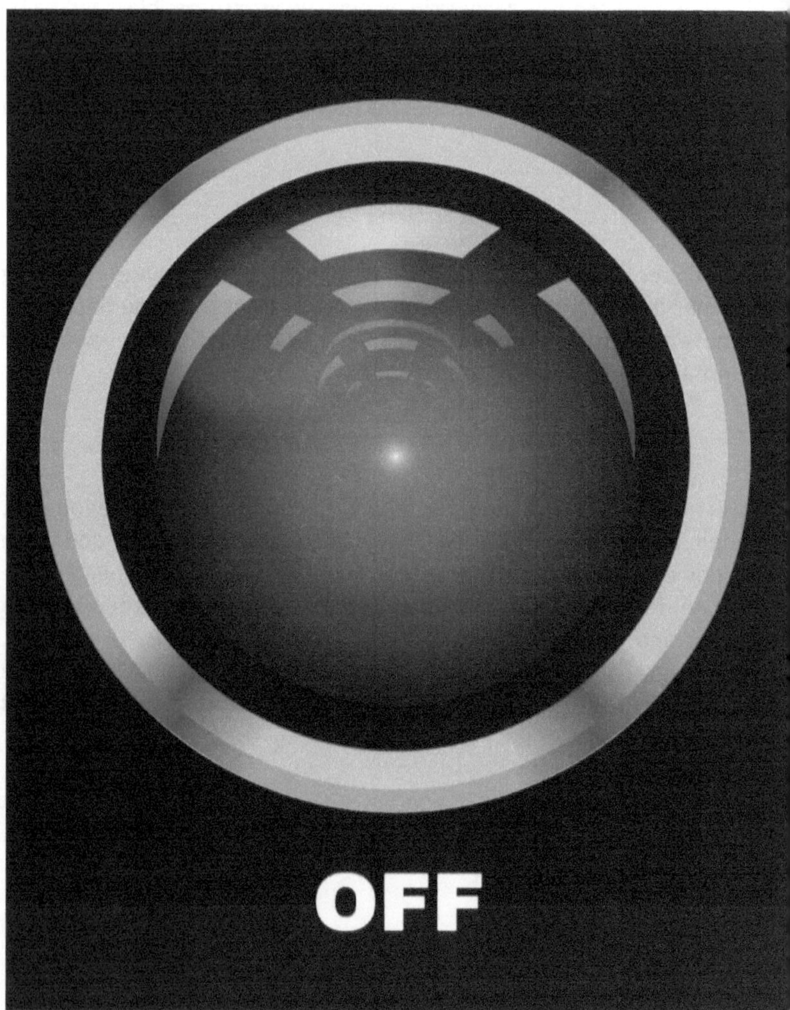

Conclusions

Time to turn off the AUTOPILOT

Humans are computers. Humans run on software created either by chance or something we have no clue about.   Humanity has been running on autopilot since the beginning. Individual humans also run on autopilot.   The human brain facilitates each separate human life and also how humans interact with each other. The brain separates humans into groups and these separations eventually causes wars that offers the rest of humanity amazing technology to propel humans as far as we need to go or maybe there is no limit.

Human emotions need to be brought under control while self-awareness needs to be increased. When self-awareness and emotions meet in the middle humanity will take the next step in our evolution.

Any type of human life is a HUMAN EXPERIENCE and there is no right or wrong life. The human consciences are a fairly new device and will be constantly changing, but up to now it has served humanity well. Eight billion living humans with technology to move humanity off planet Earth are indescribable accomplishments. We all must remember that being ALIVE is also an indescribable accomplishment.

When an individual human becomes self-aware and understands their emotions, then their life may take on a different meaning. Emotions have also served humanity well and these emotions are the core values when discussing humanity on autopilot.

Most humans just follow their emotions without a moment of self-awareness. This is living on autopilot. When a county invades another with only its self-interest at heart, this is certainly living on autopilot.

When individual humans and humanity as a whole ask the question, "What motivates us to do anything?" then the path to the next level is one step closer. The number of levels are endless, but surely humanity is ready for a new directive. The level that humanity is on now is just so yesterday and needs to change as soon as possible. When self -awareness and emotions meet in the middle, the change will be obvious.

No one can change the system by picking a side. When humans stop selecting one group over another and start selecting "humanity," then life may suddenly produce the most unexpected events that no human has ever imagined.

What motivates any human to do anything?

What motivates you to do anything?

Neutral or Better

Please sign up for the

Neutral or Better Newsletter

Please send your information to

neutralobserver77@gmail.com